The Healthy Eating Plan

Stella G McGovern

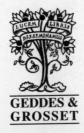

GEDDES & GROSSET

First Published 2001 by Geddes & Grosset

Text by Stella G McGovern

© 2001 Geddes & Grosset, David Dale House,
New Lanark, Scotland, ML11 9DJ

ISBN 1 84205 103 2

Printed and bound in the UK

Contents

1
Body, Mind
and Diet

II
Diets Guide

III
Your Healthy Eating and Exercise Plan

1
Body, Mind and Diet

Introduction

I N Britain, as in many other western countries, both the state of being overweight and actual obesity are reaching epidemic proportions. It is estimated that as many as 20 million people, or one in three adults, are overweight and 6 million are obese – statistics which are causing increasing concern among health professionals. The reason behind their concern is that people who are considerably overweight or obese run an increased risk of contracting a variety of serious illnesses or conditions, many of which are life-threatening. One particularly worrying trend is the increase in the number of overweight children. Heavy children often become fat adults and it is feared that these individuals could all become victim to illnesses linked to obesity at a young age; conditions which should otherwise be preventable. The potential health consequences of obesity are not only awful for the people concerned, but place an additional strain upon an over-burdened National Health Service. Hence it is perhaps not surprising that since the alarm bells began ringing several years ago over the rising levels of obesity, government-run campaigns involving the whole area of diet, nutrition and health have become increasingly prominent. People in Britain today are bombarded with information about what they should or should not eat and the lifestyle that they should aim to adopt.

Education about eating for good health forms a part of the National Curriculum and every school is expected to provide 'health foods' for its pupils. While all this information is meant to be helpful, there is some evidence that it is failing in its aims, at least among some sections of the population and, at worst, is causing worry and confusion. Young people may simply ignore the advice while those on low incomes frequently feel that they cannot afford to buy good, healthy foods. Hence it is important that any book about diets should be accessible to all and convey the message that each person should try to eat healthily and maintain a reasonable weight.

There is a difference between maintaining an acceptable weight for reasons of good health and the fashion-led obsession with dieting which

Body, Mind, and Diet

is prevalent in Britain and other western countries. Of course, the decision to diet is ultimately a matter of personal choice, but it is probably the case that, especially among the young, dieting is driven by a desire to achieve the body size which is held up to be the fashionable ideal. For many years, the fashion industry has equated extreme thinness in women with ideal beauty and this has gone hand-in-hand with an inexorable rise in the number of people affected by eating disorders (see page 48). The fashion industry has been held partly responsible for this trend. In May 2000, the British Medical Association found it responsible for promoting an ideal of female beauty which is unattainable, abnormal and unhealthy. There are now some hopeful signs that the more responsible members of the industry are taking these concerns seriously and perhaps eventually, this will result in fewer people having their lives prematurely cut short by eating disorders.

In the late 20th century, dieting itself became a multi-million pound industry with new 'miracle' diets and products claiming to promote weight loss, appearing on the market on a regular basis. The trend shows no sign of abating and it is certain that the diet industry will continue to take pounds from people's pockets as well as from their waistlines! Diet plans are discussed in this book but it should be emphasized that it is not necessary to spend a fortune in order to achieve a reduction in weight. There is no harm in trying a new diet plan or product if you wish to do so, but for many people, a sensible adjustment in eating habits can result in the achievement and maintenance of a desirable weight. A slow and steady weight loss over a period of weeks or months is considered by most experts to be the most effective method and the one which offers the best hope that the pounds will not merely pile back on again! However, there is little doubt that a whole range of psychological and emotional factors, along with individual temperament, are key factors in successful dieting and these are also discussed in this book.

It is hoped that the contents will prove equally useful and encouraging to those who are very overweight or obese and need to lose weight for health reasons, as well as to those who just wish to lose a few pounds.

Eating for Good Health – The Basics of Nutrition

IN recent years, there has been a great deal of confusion about what constitutes a healthy diet. However, it is now universally recognized that the type of western diet eaten by many people in Britain, which is high in saturated animal fat and cholesterol, salt, sugar and refined carbohydrates but low in fibre, is bad for health and is implicated in the development of several serious medical conditions. This type of diet is largely based on an over-consumption of meat, dairy products and highly processed foods, with the ill effects being compounded by lack of exercise, smoking and excess drinking of alcohol.

In contrast, health and nutritional experts recommend a wholefood diet based on foods eaten in as natural a state as possible. Before considering weight loss diets, it is useful to gain an understanding of the needs of the human body for the various nutritional elements contained in food.

The human body requires food to provide energy for all life processes and for growth, repair and maintenance of cells and tissues, including those of the immune system, brain and nervous system and other vital organs. Individual needs vary according to activity levels and age but, in general, men require proportionately more food than women due to their larger body size. Young, active people and growing children require more food than those who are elderly and sedentary. In addition, slight internal differences exist between individuals who may outwardly appear comparable.

Elements of food

There are three main groups of substances contained in food which are needed by the body in differing amounts: carbohydrates, proteins and fats. In addition, the body requires fibre (derived from plants), which is highly significant in promoting good health and in preventing a number of life-threatening diseases. Vitamins and minerals are needed in small amounts on a daily basis and these are normally supplied by eating a variety of different foods. However, supplements may be helpful for those on particularly strict, weight loss diets.

Carbohydrates

Carbohydrates are organic compounds which may be simple or complex and their role is to provide an easily utilised source of energy for the body (measured in calories). All carbohydrates are composed of carbon, hydrogen and oxygen and are manufactured by plants. The simplest forms are sugars, of which the most basic is glucose. All carbohydrates are eventually broken down by digestive processes into glucose, which is absorbed and utilised by the body in various ways. When sugars are involved, the process is rapid and the resulting glucose is soon absorbed into the bloodstream. It may then be used immediately, particularly if energy demands are high, as during vigorous exercise, and athletes often take glucose expressly for this purpose. Glucose is also required for the healthy function of red blood cells and is the main source of energy for the brain.

Starches

Starches are more complex (polysaccharide) carbohydrates, built up of chains of simple glucose molecules. They take longer to be broken down by digestive processes than sugars, so providing a slower, more gradual supply of glucose. The body fluids and blood generally contain enough reserves of glucose to meet the energy requirements for one day's activity. In conditions in which there is a lack of available glucose (as in starvation or extreme physical exercise) the body is able to manufacture it, at least for a time, in the liver by a process called gluconeogenesis. Glycerol (derived from fat stores) and amino acids (from proteins in muscle or in the diet) are used as raw materials in this process. Conversely, excess glucose is converted by the liver into the complex (polysaccharide) carbohydrate glycogen (animal starch).

This is stored in the body, particularly in liver and muscle cells and is used first when there is a lack of glucose in the blood. It is the glycogen store which is initially used up when a person embarks upon a calorie reduced diet and this is utilised quite rapidly. It is only when glycogen has been depleted that fat deposits begin to be mobilised as a source of energy.

In general, simple sugars, especially the refined type found in processed foodstuffs such as sweets, biscuits, cakes, chocolates, sauces, etc., merely provide the body with calories, usually in excess of the amount needed for energy requirements. Starches, which are found in a wide range of foods including cereals, grains, bread, pasta, potatoes and other vegetables and fruits, are far more useful and often have accompanying fibre, vitamins and minerals. However, the levels of beneficial substances are reduced in starchy foods which are processed and refined, such as white varieties of bread, pasta, flour and rice. Many people in the West eat only these unhelpful forms of refined sugars and carbohydrates which are easily eaten to excess and are readily converted into fat, greatly contributing towards the problems of weight gain and obesity. Nutritional experts recommend that complex carbohydrates in the form of starchy foods should constitute 60 to 70 per cent of the overall daily intake of calories. These should be in the form of wholemeal bread, cereals, whole grains, brown rice, pasta and potatoes (especially with their skins) which have a high content of fibre as well as starch. They are more satisfying and filling than white varieties of the same foods and hence reduce the tendency to overeat. This not only aids weight loss in obesity but assists in the maintenance of a correct and healthy weight. A good way to make such an adjustment in the diet is not to change overnight from refined to non-refined carbohydrates but to gradually replace, for example, white bread with wholemeal with the eventual aim of eating mainly unrefined, high fibre foods.

Proteins

Proteins are the structural components of the body forming the basis of cells, tissues and organs. They are a large group of organic compounds consisting of carbon, hydrogen, nitrogen and oxygen atoms. These are arranged in various ways to form units called amino acids which, when joined together in long chains, make up the structure of the protein. There are 20 basic amino acids which are usually arranged in linear molecules known as polypeptides. Although there are only 20 different kinds, there are a huge number of possible arrangements in a polypeptide or protein, as the amino acids can be in any order. Most proteins consist of more than one polypeptide chain and there are many thousands of them in the human body, each with a unique structure but all made from the 'pool' of 20 amino acids. In addition to being structural molecules, proteins are a vital component of chromosomes (genetic material) and are used in the body for storage, as messengers (e.g. hormones), as carriers (e.g. the globin in the haemoglobin of blood which transports oxygen) and as catalysts of metabolic, biochemical reactions (enzymes).

The body is capable of manufacturing 12 of the 20 basic amino acids. However, the remainder, called the 'essential amino acids' must be obtained from food. Hence it is important for anyone embarking upon a weight loss diet to include some protein among the foods that are eaten. Proteins are widely found in foods derived both from plant and animal sources. Plant sources include beans, peas, pulses, whole grains, nuts and seeds while red meat, liver, kidney, poultry, fish, milk, cheese and dairy produce are the principal animal sources. Red meat is a good source of essential amino acids and iron and is traditionally regarded as 'first class' protein. However, there are plenty of other protein-rich foods and vegetarians can choose from dairy products and plant sources. It is generally recommended that the consumption of red meat should be limited to once or twice a week with chicken, fish, pulses, beans, etc., which are high in protein but low in saturated fat, chosen as alternatives. Also, proteins should make up about 15 to 20 per cent of the daily diet (although this figure is a contentious one).

In Britain, the average consumption of protein constitutes about 40 per cent of daily calorie intake and it is often eaten at the expense of other foods such as green vegetables or cereals. Oily fish (e.g. mackerel, herring, sardines, salmon, trout) are good sources both of protein and essential unsaturated oils which help to prevent the development of heart disease. It is generally recommended by nutritional experts that oily fish should be eaten two or three times each week. Peas and beans, which are good sources of vegetable protein, are additionally beneficial as they can act to reduce levels of blood cholesterol (see also fats below).

Proteins are essential throughout life for repair and replacement of damaged cells and tissues. However, it is particularly important for growing children to receive plenty of protein in their diet since they are laying down the foundations of bones and muscles which must last for a lifetime. Inadequate protein in the diet (rare in western countries but see Eating Disorders, page 48) soon shows externally in dull, lacklustre hair, skin and nails, but, internally, the body's metabolic processes may be breaking down muscle tissue to effect essential 'repairs' elsewhere. Hence no weight loss diet should be devoid of protein, particularly if a person is to stay on it for any length of time.

Fats
Fats are a group of organic compounds that occur naturally in plant and animal cells in the form of lipids, consisting of carbon, hydrogen and oxygen

atoms. Lipids include oils, fats, waxes and related substances known as 'derived lipids'. A fat consists of one glycerol and three fatty acid molecules, collectively known as a triglyceride, and during digestion, is broken down into its constituent parts by enzymes called lipases. Fats play a vital role in the human body and perform many functions. They are an important energy store, having twice the calorific value (38 calories per gram) of carbohydrates. In human beings, fat is deposited in a layer beneath the skin (subcutaneous fat) where it provides cushioning and insulation. This fat includes the 'cellulite' which is public enemy number one of the diet industry! In fact, it is nothing more than plain fat and no different to other forms of fat elsewhere. Fat is also laid down in deeper regions of the body, within cells and around organs, where it is known as 'adipose tissue'. All animal fat is solid at room temperature and is of the type known as saturated fat (see below).

Human beings are designed to store fat as an energy store, with women carrying a greater proportion (22 per cent of body weight) than men (15 per cent). The difference is reflected in the fact that women have many more fat cells than men (about 35 billion compared to 28 billion in men). Female fat reserves are present so that they can be utilised during pregnancy, particularly during conditions of food shortage. From an evolutionary standpoint, this makes sound biological sense conferring a greater chance that mother and infant will survive. It is particularly unfortunate that the natural female tendency to store a certain proportion of fat should have become something which is regarded as so unacceptable to those who set the style and fashion of today.

In modern discussions about diet, a great deal is heard about saturated and unsaturated fat. Whether a fat is saturated or unsaturated depends upon its chemical properties. Saturated fats have all their available chemical bonds filled with hydrogen atoms and cannot join with other compounds. Unsaturated fats do not have the full complement of hydrogen atoms in their structure and this gives them a softer and more liquid consistency. Fatty acids have three major functions in the human body:

1 They are the building blocks of phospholipids (lipids containing phosphate) and glycolipids (lipids containing carbohydrate). These molecules are vital components of the outer, surrounding membranes of all cells, controlling the passage of substances both inwards and outwards and hence are vital to the functioning of the body at cellular level.

2 Fatty acid derivatives, i.e. compounds that are made from fatty acids, serve as hormones and chemical messengers within and between cells.

3 Fatty acids are stored within cells as triglycerides (i.e. joined to glycerol molecules) as fuel reserves. They are broken down when required to release large quantities of energy.

Saturated fats, e.g. cholesterol, are found in meat and dairy products such as whole milk, cheese, butter and eggs. Many processed foods have saturated fats added to them and they are widely used in food manufacturing. Saturated fatty acids are converted by liver cells into cholesterol, which is a vital substance in the body, being a component of cell membranes and a precursor or stage in the production of steroid hormones (e.g. the sex hormones) and of bile salts. However, an excess level in the blood causes atheroma or furring of the arteries, which is a causal factor in angina, strokes and various forms of heart disease and is implicated in diabetes mellitus. Men and post-menopausal women in western countries are at particular risk of premature death from strokes and heart disease. Of course, an excess of cholesterol and saturated fat in the diet is also linked to weight gain and obesity. It has been established beyond doubt that there is a definite link between consumption of a western diet, rich in saturated fat, obesity and high incidence of heart disease.

Unsaturated fats or oils are of two types: polyunsaturated and monounsaturated. Monounsaturated fats have one available site in the molecule to bind to a hydrogen atom. Sources include olive oil, rapeseed oil, groundnut oil and some fish oils. Polyunsaturated fats have several available sites for binding to hydrogen atoms in their molecular structure. Sources include oily fish (e.g. mackerel, salmon, herring, trout), vegetable oils (e.g. corn, sunflower, safflower, rapeseed) and nuts and seeds such as walnuts and sesame seeds. Among the polyunsaturated group are those called the 'essential fatty acids' which human beings can only obtain from food. These must be included in the diet to ensure good health, highlighting the fact that any weight loss programme should ideally allow for the eating of a small amount of fat. Important essential fatty acids include linoleic and linolenic acid, which have been shown to lower the levels of triglycerides and cholesterol in the blood and decrease the tendency for clotting factors called platelets to clump together. High blood levels of cholesterol and triglycerides and aggregation of platelets are all involved in the development of furred, blocked arteries and heart disease. Good sources of linoleic acids are soya, safflower, sunflower, corn and walnut oil. Good sources of linolenic acid are linseed, flaxseed, walnut and soya oils. Another essential fatty acid is eicosapentaenoic acid or EPA and this is also protective against heart disease. A good source is oily fish such as the types listed on page 16.

Human blood contains substances called lipoproteins which are molecules of protein that carry fat. These are of two types: low density lipoproteins (LDL) and high-density lipoproteins (HDL). The relative ratio of LDL to HDL is crucial in the prevention or development of arterial disease. This is because HDL caries cholesterol to the liver where it is broken down and eventually eliminated. However, LDL deposits cholesterol and so platelets are encouraged to aggregate which leads to narrowing of the arterial lumen (internal space), allowing fat deposits to be trapped resulting in furring of the arteries. Linoleic and linolenic acids and EPA inhibit the clumping together of platelets. Studies have shown that people who naturally eat a diet rich in fish oils, such as the Japanese and Inuit (Eskimo) people, have very little heart disease. It is only if they change to the western type of diet, rich in saturated animal fat and cholesterol, that their incidence of heart disease increases.

Hence, for those who are not vegetarians, it is recommended that oily fish is eaten two or three times each week and, ideally, it should be possible to incorporate this into a sensible weight loss diet. It is the overall ratio of HDL to LDL that is important, with the aim of keeping blood cholesterol at a low level. Other recommendations might therefore include using skimmed or semi-skimmed milk, eating low fat dairy products (cottage cheese, some yoghurts, fat-reduced cheese), choosing chicken or white fish and grilling or steaming, rather than frying, food. In addition, it is advisable to eat red meat sparingly, to limit the consumption of eggs to no more than two each week and to cut down on processed meats and foods. The healthy vegetable oils mentioned above can be used in cooking and, since the human body is able to convert linolenic acid into EPA, vegetarians are able to choose alternatives to oily fish. The richest source of linolenic acid is flaxseed oil which also contains useful amounts of linoleic acid. EPA from fish oils and linolenic acid from flaxseed or linseed oil have the additional advantage of having anti-allergic and anti-inflammatory properties. Eczema, psoriasis, rheumatoid arthritis and menstrual symptoms are all conditions that have shown improvement in some people when intake of these oils has been increased.

The general recommendation for a healthy diet is that fat should constitute 30 per cent or less of the total intake of calories and that it should largely be of the beneficial polyunsaturated forms listed on page 16. From this discussion, it can be seen that eating this type of fat not only safeguards health but also should not hinder achieving and maintaining a sensible weight.

Fibre

Fibre is derived from the cell walls of plants. In recent years, the absence of sufficient quantities of dietary fibre has been recognized as one of the most significant causes of ill-health, particularly in western countries. Not only is a lack of dietary fibre implicated in the incidence of a number of serious conditions, but it is also very much part of the equation with regard to obesity. People who eat a largely plant-based, high fibre diet are far less likely to suffer from diseases such as bowel cancer and are rarely overweight or obese. However, if the same people change to a western diet that is low in dietary fibre, these conditions begin to appear. Dietary fibre, also known as roughage, has various components, the most significant of which is cellulose which forms the main part of plant cell walls. The most readily available sources are foods containing wholewheat bran, such as wholemeal flour and bread, brown varieties of rice, pasta and spaghetti. Cellulose cannot be digested directly by the human gut, although a certain amount of degradation is brought about by the natural population of bacteria in the colon. Cellulose is insoluble fibre, i.e. it does not break down in water. It is able to bind to water and promotes healthy and regular bowel function. The other components of fibre are termed non-cellulose complex polysaccharides, i.e. they are carbohydrates.

Pectins are found in many fruits and peel, especially citrus rinds and in vegetables and their skins. They have gel-producing effects and are able to bind to cholesterol and bile salts in the intestine so that these substances are eliminated rather than absorbed. Pectins are water soluble and promote a slower release of food from the stomach and a longer time for beneficial nutrients to be absorbed. This has the effect of helping to prevent a sudden after-meal elevation in blood sugar, something which is particularly important for people with diabetes. Hemicelluloses are found in oat bran, seeds, peas and beans, grains, vegetables and fruit. They are an important

18

source of helpful short-chain fatty acids which provide energy for the cells in the lining of the colon and are believed to have anti-cancer properties. Eating oats, e.g. as porridge, has been shown to lower blood cholesterol levels and hence reduce the risk of atherosclerosis and heart disease. Mucilages are found in seeds and beans and one type, guar gum, is widely used commercially in both food and non-food products. Mucilages remove cholesterol, delay the emptying of the stomach and reduce after-meal peaks of blood glucose and insulin, again important in diabetes. They also act as natural laxatives. Gums, like pectins, are gel-forming substances and are soluble in water. One form, gum arabic, is widely used by the food industry and also acts as a natural laxative. Lignins are fibres that are found especially in the woody parts of plants but also in vegetables, fruits and grains. They possess anti-microbial and anti-cancer properties. Algal fibre is primarily obtained from seaweeds and two well-known examples, agar and carrageenan, are widely used in food manufacturing.

The beneficial effects of eating a range of dietary fibre are well established and can be summarised as follows:

1   The presence of fibre necessitates a more thorough chewing of food and hence slows down eating – one of the practices recommended for those on a diet. This produces a more rapid feeling of fullness and so there is less likelihood of overeating and weight gain. This is helpful to someone who is trying to lose weight since it means that a feeling of satisfaction can be obtained from a smaller intake of food.

2   A high proportion of fibre delays the passage of food from the stomach into the intestine so that this becomes a gradual process. This reduces the 'peaking' of blood sugar levels that tends to occur after meals, resulting in a lower rise and a more prolonged provision of energy. This is very important in both the prevention and treatment of diabetes mellitus because of the effect on blood glucose and hence on the release of insulin.

3   Fibre in the diet promotes a greater release of enzymes, hormones and secretions from the pancreas, which are vital for digestion, and hence encourages an effective digestive process. It is important for anyone on a diet, or who is 'weight watching', to ensure that they receive the

full nutritional benefit from the food that is being eaten and the inclusion of fibre helps to make sure that this is the case.

4   A high intake of soluble fibre removes cholesterol and triglycerides from the blood and promotes their elimination. This is not only enormously beneficial in preventing heart and circulatory disease but lessens the possibility of these substances being deposited as fat.

5   A high fibre diet promotes healthy bowel function and reduces the likelihood of constipation and the development of haemorrhoids and diverticulitis.

6   Dietary fibre favours the growth of helpful acid-loving bacteria in the colon at the expense of harmful species that produce endotoxins. These acid-loving bacteria are able to partially ferment the digested food, providing the body with useful short-chain fatty acids utilised by the liver, as well as energy which is available to the cells lining the colon. The short-chain fatty acids, particularly butyrate, have been shown to possess anti-carcinogenic properties.

Cautionary note: particular forms of fibre may not be helpful for people suffering from certain digestive complaints or conditions. In older age, too much fibre or particular types of fibre, may cause symptoms of 'wind' or an upset stomach and in these circumstances, it is best to exercise caution. Wheat bran is one form of fibre which seems to cause problems for some people. By trial and error, it is usually possible to establish the types of high fibre foods which are causing problems and to substitute alternatives. Obviously, a high fibre, weight-loss diet is unlikely to be suitable for someone who suffers from these types of problems!

The general recommendation is that healthy adults should try to eat about 30 g (10 oz) of fibre each day. This is easily achieved by eating fibre-containing breakfast cereals, wholemeal bread, brown rice and pasta, fruits, vegetables and salads (at least five portions from the last three every day) and pulses (lentils, beans, peas, etc.).

Vitamins

Vitamins are a group of organic substances that are required in minute quantities in the diet to maintain good health. They are involved in a large number of cellular processes, including growth and repair of tissues and organs, metabolism of food and functioning of the immune, nervous, circulatory and hormonal systems.

There are two groups of vitamins: those that are fat-soluble, including A, D, E and K and those that are water-soluble – C (ascorbic acid) and the B group. A lack of a particular vitamin may result in a deficiency disease – a condition which is fortunately rare in western countries although those following a strict dietary regime may be at risk! Water-soluble vitamins dissolve in water and cannot be stored in the body so they must be obtained from the diet on a daily basis. Any excess is simply excreted. Fat-soluble vitamins (with the partial exception of D and K) are also obtained from food, but any excess can be stored by the liver. Hence they are needed on a regular basis in order to maintain the body's reserves. However, excessive doses, particularly of A and D (usually as a result of taking too many supplements), can have toxic effects because of a build-up in the liver.

An examination of the role of each vitamin is valuable for the would-be dieter as it helps to explain the importance of including these nutrients in the dietary plan that is adopted.

Vitamin A

Vitamin A (retinol) is a fat-soluble vitamin that must be obtained from the diet. It has a vital role in maintaining the epithelial layers of the skin and mucous membranes so that these function effectively and produce their secretions. It is also needed for the manufacture of rhodopsin, also called 'visual purple', a light-sensitive pigment that is essential for vision in dim light. Good sources of vitamin A are orange and yellow vegetables and fruits, particularly carrots, peaches and apricots and also green vegetables, eggs, dairy products (full fat), liver and fish oils. Vegetables, especially carrots, contain plant substances called carotenes or carotenoids, some of which are precursors of vitamin A, i.e. they can be converted into the vitamin. Carotenes such as beta-carotene also have vital antioxidant properties, as does vitamin A itself. Due to its role in maintaining the health of the body's epithelial surfaces, vitamin A has also been shown to enhance the immune response by boosting the cells that fight infections and tumours. Deficiency of vitamin A causes night blindness and a deterioration in the health of mucous membranes and skin. This can cause increased respiratory and ear infections, dry skin and a greater susceptibility to skin conditions and dull, lifeless hair. A sustained lack of vitamin A contributes to the failure of a child to grow and thrive, and weight loss and general debility in adults. The RDA (recommended daily amount) is 0.75 mg but excessive doses should be avoided as these can cause toxic effects.

Vitamin B_1

Vitamin B_1 (thiamine or aneurine) is involved in carbohydrate metabolism and the vital provision of energy for all body processes. It is essential for the healthy functioning of the nervous system and muscles and is a water-soluble vitamin. It plays a part in the mechanisms that combat pain and it may have a role in the intellectual functions of the brain. Good sources of vitamin B_1 are whole grains, potatoes, brown rice, yeast, pulses, green vegetables, eggs, dairy products, liver, kidney, meat, chicken and fish. A slight deficiency causes digestive upset, sickness, constipation, tiredness, irritability and forgetfulness. Prolonged lack of thiamine causes the development of the deficiency disease, beri beri, which occurs mainly in countries in which the staple diet is polished rice. This causes inflammation of nerves and results in fever, breathing difficulties, palpitations and possible heart failure and death. The RDA is 1 to 1.3 mg.

Vitamin B_2

Vitamin B_2 (riboflavin) is involved in carbohydrate metabolism in the enzyme reactions within cells and hence in the provision of energy. It also helps to maintain the health of the mucous membranes and skin. It is a water-soluble vitamin that must be obtained from food, with similar sources to those for thiamine. A deficiency may cause a sore, irritated tongue and lips, dry skin and scalp and possibly, nervousness, trembling, sleeplessness and giddiness. The RDA is 1.3 to 1.6 mg.

Vitamin B_3

Vitamin B_3 (niacin, nicotinic acid) is involved in the maintenance of healthy blood and circulation, the nervous system and the functioning of the adrenal glands. It is a water-soluble vitamin and good sources include some cereals (excluding maize), peanuts, beans, dried fruits, globe artichokes, meat, kidney, liver and chicken. A deficiency causes sickness and diarrhoea, appetite loss, peptic ulcers, dermatitis, irritability, depression, sleeplessness, headaches and tiredness. In more severe cases, the deficiency disease pellagra arises producing the symptoms listed above but with accompanying dementia. Pellagra usually arises in people eating a diet based on maize with an associated lack of animal protein or dairy products. Although maize contains nicotinic acid, it is in an unusable form and does not contain the essential amino acid tryptophan, which the body needs to utilise the acid. The RDA is 1.8 mg.

Vitamin B_5

Vitamin B_5 (pantothenic acid) is involved in the metabolism of carbohydrates and fats and in the maintenance of the nervous and immune systems, as well as in the function of the adrenal glands. It is widely found in all types of food and is also produced within the gut. Deficiency is uncommon but low levels may be associated with poor adrenal gland function (causing headaches, tiredness, sleeplessness, sickness and abdominal pains), particularly at times of stress. The RDA is 4 to 7 mg.

Vitamin B_6

Vitamin B_6 (pyroxidine) is involved in the metabolism of certain amino acids and in the functioning of the immune system in its production of antibodies to combat infection. It is involved in the manufacture of red blood cells and in the metabolism of carbohydrates and fats. It is a water-soluble vitamin that is widely found in many foods. A deficiency may play a role in the development of atherosclerosis and depression of the immune system. The RDA is 1.5 to 2 mg.

Vitamin B_9

Vitamin B_9 (folic acid) is necessary for the correct functioning of vitamin B_{12} in the production of red blood cells and in the metabolism of carbohydrates, fats and proteins. It is a water-soluble vitamin and good sources include liver, kidney, green vegetables, yeast, fruits, dried beans and pulses, whole grains and wheatgerm. A deficiency in folic acid is quite common and produces anaemia tiredness, sleeplessness, forgetfulness and irritability. A good intake of folic acid is important for women trying to conceive and in maintaining a healthy pregnancy. A deficiency in folic acid is a common finding in women with cervical dysplasia (abnormality in cells of the cervix, which can be a precancerous condition) and in those taking oral contraceptives. In addition, it is commonly deficient in people suffering from some forms of mental illness, depression, Crohn's disease and ulcerative colitis.

Elderly people are quite frequently found to have low levels of folic acid. The RDA is 0.3 mg.

Vitamin B₁₂

Vitamin B_{12} (cyanocobalamin) is necessary for the correct functioning of folic acid and is important in the production of nucleic acids (genetic material). Also in the maintenance of the myelin (fatty) sheath surrounding nerve fibres, without which they cannot function, and in the production of red blood cells. It is involved in the metabolism of proteins, carbohydrates and fats and in the maintenance of healthy cells. It is a water-soluble vitamin that is found in dairy products, egg yolks, meat, liver, kidney and fish. Blood levels of vitamin B_{12} are often low in people suffering from Alzheimer's disease and some other psychiatric disorders. Deficiency results in anaemia, but often this is the result of faulty absorption of the vitamin rather than dietary lack. In order for the vitamin to be absorbed, a substance known as 'intrinsic factor' must be produced, along with hydrochloric acid by the secretory cells in the stomach. When this mechanism is defective, the condition known as pernicious anaemia may arise. Prolonged B_{12} deficiency causes severe degeneration of the nervous system, producing symptoms of tingling and numbness in the limbs, loss of certain reflexes and sensations, lack of coordination, speech difficulties, confusion, irritability and depression. In addition, there is pallor, tiredness, breathlessness and irregular heartbeat caused by the development of anaemia. The RDA is 2 micrograms (0.02 mg).

Biotin

Biotin (vitamin B complex) is a water-soluble vitamin involved in the metabolism of fats, including the production of glucose in conditions in which there is a lack of available carbohydrates. It works in conjunction (although independently) with insulin and can be important in the treatment of diabetes. Good sources of biotin include egg yolk, liver, kidney, wheat, oats, yeast and nuts, and it is also synthesized by gut bacteria. Deficiency is very uncommon in adults but in young infants a lack of biotin may be a cause of seborrhoeic dermatitis (cradle cap). The RDA is 0.1 to 0.2 mg.

Vitamin C

Vitamin C (ascorbic acid) is an extremely important nutrient, vital in the maintenance of cell walls and connective tissue and essential for the health of blood vessels, cartilage, gums, skin, tendons and ligaments. It facilitates the uptake and absorption of iron, is involved in the immune system in fighting off infections and has anti-viral properties. It also promotes the repair of wounds and has vital antioxidant activity. It is important in the correct functioning of the adrenal glands, especially at times of stress. Blood levels of vitamin C are often low in people suffering from asthma. Since it is involved in the metabolism of fats and the control of cholesterol, a dietary lack of vitamin C is significant in the development of atherosclerosis. The levels of vitamin C in the lens and fluid of the eye is low in people with cataracts. This is also the case in women with cervical dysplasia (abnormal cells in the neck of the womb) and people suffering from Crohn's disease or fistula (an abnormal opening between two hollow organs or between such an organ or gland and the exterior). A study of men with hypertension (high blood pressure) revealed that they also had low blood levels of vitamin C.

Due to its effects on cartilage and connective tissue, lack of the vitamin is thought to be a contributory factor in the development and progression of osteoarthritis. Likewise, vitamin C is vital in the prevention of gum disease and in the repair of tendons, ligaments and connective tissue. It is water-soluble and is found in fresh fruits (especially citrus and red and black berries) and vegetables. A deficiency causes the development of scurvy, the symptoms of which include swollen, bleeding gums and loosened teeth, bleeding beneath the skin, numerous infections, tiredness, loss of muscle mass and weakness, bleeding into joints, ulcers, anaemia, fainting and diarrhoea. Eventually, the major organs are affected and scurvy is ultimately fatal if not treated – a common cause of death among sailors in past centuries. Although the condition is rare in western countries, it does occasionally arise in mild form among those eating an inadequate diet. The RDA is 30 mg.

Vitamin D

Vitamin D occurs as two steroid derivatives: D_2 (calciferol) in yeast and D_3 (cholecalciferol) which is produced in the skin in the presence of sunlight. Vitamin D is vital in the control of blood calcium levels, prompting an increased absorption of the mineral from the intestine so that there is a good supply for the production and repair of bones and teeth. In addition, vitamin D promotes the uptake of phosphorus. Good dietary sources of fat-soluble vitamin D are oily fish (mackerel, sardines, salmon, tuna, kippers), liver, egg yolk, fortified margarine and dairy produce. In addition, it is produced in the skin by the action of sunlight on a form of cholesterol. Vitamin D is converted by the liver and kidneys into a much stronger form but certain diseases of these organs can reduce the effective potency of the vitamin, even when dietary levels are adequate.

In osteoporosis, it appears that the conversion process by the kidneys can be impaired although the reasons for this are not completely clear. Deficiency in vitamin D is also quite common in people suffering from Crohn's disease and ulcerative colitis. A slight deficiency in vitamin D causes tooth decay, softening of the bones with consequent risk of injury, muscular cramps and weakness. More serious deprivation causes the deficiency disease rickets in children and osteomalacia in adults. These conditions are characterised by soft bones that bend out of shape causing deformity. The condition is particularly severe in children and may result in poor, stunted growth but it is uncommon in western countries since many foods are fortified with the vitamin. The RDA is 10 micrograms (0.1 mg) and excessive doses should be avoided as these can have toxic effects.

Vitamin E
Vitamin E comprises a group of fat-soluble compounds called tocopherols, which are widely found in many foods. These are involved in sustaining the health of cell membranes and preventing damage and may be important in combating the process of ageing. Vitamin E helps to maintain the blood and skin and aids resistance to infection. Deficiency is rare in human beings but if it does occur, may cause unhealthy skin and hair and be a factor in miscarriage and in prostate gland enlargement in men. The RDA is 10 mg.

Vitamin K
Vitamin K, or menadione, is fat-soluble and is essential for the clotting of blood, being involved in the formation of prothrombin which, with calcium, is changed into thrombin during the coagulation process. The vitamin is manufactured by bacteria in the large intestine but is also found in liver, kidney, green vegetables, eggs, wholewheat and cereals. Deficiency is rare in healthy people, but has been reported in those suffering from ulcerative colitis and Crohn's disease. Rarely, it may occur if antibiotics have to be taken for a prolonged period and symptoms include nosebleeds and subcutaneous bleeding. The RDA is 70 to 140 mg.

Minerals and trace elements

Minerals are chemical substances that are generally associated with non-living materials such as rocks and metals. However, forms of them are also found in all living things and they play a vital part in many metabolic processes. Some minerals, notably calcium and phosphorus, are present in significant amounts in the human body, mainly in bones and teeth. Others, for example iron, iodine and sodium, occur in extremely small quantities but are, nonetheless, very important substances within the body.

Minerals that are needed only in minute amounts are called trace elements. As with vitamins, a lack of a particular mineral can lead to a deficiency disease with the appearance of a set of symptoms that may develop over a long period of time. The effects of deficiency may be quite complex in some cases and, as with vitamins, the condition may arise either as a direct result of dietary insufficiency or be because of some malabsorption or other dysfunction within the body.

Sodium

Sodium is essential in minute quantities to ensure the correct functioning of nerves and as a vital constituent of cellular and tissue fluids. However, the quantity required is very small and is readily obtained from eating a balanced and varied diet. Most foods contain traces of sodium, usually in the form of sodium chloride or common salt. The type of diet eaten in western countries, which frequently includes considerable amounts of processed and manufactured foods, is excessively high in salt which can contribute towards a number of serious health problems.

These include high blood pressure or hypertension, heart and circulatory disorders and strain on the kidneys, which can lead to the development of kidney disease. In order to avoid these dangers, no salt should be added to food either during cooking or at the table. It should also be remembered that almost all manufactured and processed foods have a high salt content and, if they are to be used, it is worth trying to choose low salt varieties whenever possible. Many people (and animals also) enjoy the taste of salt which can enhance the flavour of food and also acts as a preservative. However, the taste for salt is an acquired habit which can be broken and herbs and spices can be substituted to add flavour and interest to cooking. Salt substitutes, which have a higher content of potassium, are also available but people with certain disorders, including forms of heart disease, should seek medical advice before using them. Eating an occasional salty meal should not harm a healthy person but strain on the kidneys can be lessened if several glasses of water are drunk as well.

The RDA for sodium in the form of salt is 0.5 to 1.6 g. Studies have shown that the average person in a western country consumes at least twice this amount and this is a contributory factor in the incidence of the diseases mentioned on page 27. Eating wholefoods and avoiding processed ones as much as possible is a good way of reducing sodium intake.

Potassium
Potassium is a vital component of cell and tissue fluids, helping to maintain the electrolyte/water balance and it is also essential for nerve function. The balance between potassium and sodium levels in the body may be quite significant in the development of some diseases and conditions. For example, low potassium/high sodium ratios are a factor in the development of hypertension (high blood pressure) and stress. Potassium levels are usually quite high in many wholefoods but are often reduced in highly processed ones. A deficiency in potassium causes appetite loss and sickness, bloating, weakness of muscles, increased thirst, a tingling sensation and pins and needles. Blood pressure falls, which may lead to light-headedness and, in severe cases, unconsciousness and coma. In general, sufficient potassium can be obtained from eating a normal, varied diet and the RDA is 1875 to 5625 mg. Enriched potassium supplements should not be taken by people suffering from heart disorders without first obtaining medical advice.

Calcium
Calcium is present in significant amounts in the human body, forming about 2 per cent of total mass and overwhelmingly concentrated in the bones and teeth. Calcium is vital for the growth and repair of the teeth and skeleton and is particularly important for growing children and pregnant and post-menopausal women. The uptake and hence utilisation of calcium is controlled by vitamin D, but the mineral must first be broken down by stomach acid into a form that can be used. Hence, in the development and progression of some diseases, there may not be a straightforward relationship between dietary intake of calcium and what happens within the body. For example, patients with osteoporosis quite frequently have low levels of both stomach acid and the most potent

form of vitamin D, but adequate intake of calcium. Those suffering from Crohn's disease or irritable bowel syndrome may also go short of calcium as a result of vitamin deficiency, among other factors. Howver, some people suffering from high blood pressure (hypertension) have been shown to have a lower than normal dietary intake of calcium.

Calcium supplements are readily available but they are often in the form of insoluble calcium carbonate, which is less easily absorbed by the body. The most useful forms are as ionised, soluble calcium citrate, gluconate or lactate which are more readily utilised. Calcium deficiency is rare in people eating a normal, varied diet and good sources of the mineral include milk, dairy products, fish, flour, bread and fortified cereals. Severe deficiency results in rickets in children and osteomalacia in adults. People requiring extra calcium can normally obtain it from the diet but supplements may sometimes be needed. The RDA is 500 mg.

Iron

Iron is an essential component of haemoglobin, the respiratory substance in red blood cells which picks up and transports oxygen from the lungs to all the body tissues. It consists of haem, a compound containing iron composed of a pigment known as a porphyrin, which confers the red colour of the blood. This combines with the protein globin to perform the vital task of transporting oxygen from the lungs to the tissues and carbon dioxide in the reverse direction so that the latter can be eliminated from the body. Iron-rich foods include red meat, liver, kidney, egg yolk, cocoa, nuts, green vegetables, especially spinach, dried figs, apricots, raisins, pulses, fortified flour and cereals. Iron is absorbed more readily from meat but its uptake is also enhanced by plenty of vitamin C. A deficiency in iron causes anaemia with symptoms of tiredness, feeling cold, shortness of breath, dizziness and possible loss of appetite and weight, swelling of the ankles and heartbeat irregularities. Anaemia may also result from diseases or disorders of the blood or other organs rather than an actual dietary lack of iron. It is common in people suffering from leukaemia, Crohn's disease or ulcerative colitis, bleeding disorders, immune system disruption or in those who have suffered blood loss. Pregnant women and women who have just given birth are also at risk of iron deficiency. The RDA is 800 mg.

Phosphorus

Phosphorus is present in the body in considerable amounts, making up about 1 per cent of total body weight and concentrated mainly in the bones and teeth. It is essential for the growth, health and maintenance of the teeth and skeleton and the body's supply is totally renewed over two to three years. Phosphorus is also essential in energy metabolism and muscle activity and in the function of some enzymes. It is also required in the intestine for the absorption of certain other elements and compounds. A deficiency in phosphorus is unlikely as it is widely found in foods and it is present in particularly high concentrations in protein foods of animal origin. Symptoms of deficiency can include muscle and central nervous system disorders, weakness, malaise, anorexia and respiratory failure (in extreme cases). An elevated intake of phosphorus, associated with a western diet high in meat and dairy produce, eaten at the expense of plant-based foods, can reduce or prevent the absorption of iron, calcium, zinc and magnesium. This may be a factor in the incidence of osteoporosis and a number of other disorders. The RDA is 800 mg.

Magnesium

Magnesium is required for the growth, health and maintenance of bones and teeth, the correct functioning of nerves and muscles, and for metabolic processes involving certain enzymes. It is also involved in the functioning of vitamins B_1 and B_{12}. Magnesium is widely found in many foods, including green vegetables, cereals, whole grains, milk, dairy products, eggs, shellfish, nuts and pulses. A deficiency causes anxiety, sleeplessness, trembling, palpitations, cramp-like muscle pains, sickness, and loss of appetite and weight. It may be a feature in premenstrual syndrome, low blood sugar (hypoglycaemia), angina pectoris, heart attack, Crohn's disease, ulcerative colitis, diabetes mellitus, retinopathy (eye disease), hypertension, kidney stones, prolapse of the mitral valve of the heart, migraine and osteoporosis. The RDA is 300 mg.

Iodine

Iodine is vital for the correct functioning of the thyroid gland and is present in the hormones thyroxine and triiodothyronine that are essential for the regulation of metabolism and growth. Iodine is present in seafoods, seaweed, sea salt, meat and vegetables and fruits grown on iodine-rich soils. A deficiency causes goitre, in which the thyroid gland enlarges in order to increase its output of hormones. Symptoms include tiredness, lowered metabolism, weakness and weight gain. Iodine deficiency, combined with hypothyroidism (reduced thyroid activity), may be associated with fibrocystic disease of the breast and even breast cancer (in some cases). The RDA is 0.14 to 0.15 mg but this amount is greatly exceeded in the average western diet.

Zinc

Zinc is essential for the functioning of numerous enzymes and is widely involved in metabolic processes. It is vital in vitamin A utilisation, essential in immune system functioning, acts as an antioxidant and antiviral agent, and promotes the healing of wounds. It is vital for insulin metabolism and hence the control of blood sugar. Deficiency has wide-ranging effects, such as poor growth and development (including retardation of sexual and intellectual functions) in children and slow healing of wounds. Zinc deficiency is common in people suffering from Crohn's disease, hypothyroidism and gum disease and probably plays a part in susceptibility to viral infections and diabetes mellitus. The RDA is 1.5 mg.

Selenium

Selenium, in conjunction with vitamin E, is a powerful antioxidant, being the co-factor necessary for the activity of the enzyme glutathione peroxidase which mops up free radicals. Selenium ensures correct functioning of the liver and blood system but it is believed that many people are deficient in this mineral. Good sources of selenium include unrefined wholefoods such as grains and cereals, egg yolks, kidney, liver, shellfish, garlic and yeast. A deficiency in selenium can cause effects on the heart and circulation and may be implicated in some cases of anaemia. The RDA is 0.05 to 0.2 mg.

Manganese

Manganese is essential for the activity of many enzymes and metabolic reactions. It is involved in nerve and muscle function, in growth and in the health and maintenance of the skeleton. It is a co-factor in a vital enzyme of glucose metabolism and some people suffering from diabetes mellitus have been shown to be deficient in manganese. The mineral is necessary for the activity of an enzyme which has important antioxidant activity and one which is sometimes deficient in people suffering from rheumatoid arthritis. Adequate intake of manganese may be helpful in preventing and treating this condition. Manganese is widely found in many foods but especially in whole grains, nuts, cereals, avocado pears, pulses and tea. A deficiency causes slow growth and bone abnormalities. An excess can be equally damaging causing learning difficulties and central nervous system effects. The RDA is 2.5 mg.

Copper

Copper is involved in the activity of many enzymes and metabolic functions. It is necessary for the growth and maintenance of bones and is involved in the production of red blood cells. It is involved in the production of connective tissue and in the metabolism of fats, and deficiency may be a factor in the development of atherosclerosis and osteoarthritis. The zinc-copper balance has been shown to be important in the development of some conditions as the two minerals may 'compete' with one another to a certain extent. A deficiency in copper is normally uncommon but can cause reduced numbers of white blood cells, hence lowered immunity and also changes in the hair. An excessive intake of copper is also harmful and may be involved in causing joint damage, learning difficulties and increased susceptibility to gum disease.

Chromium

Chromium is important in a range of metabolic activities, particularly the utilisation and storage of sugars and fats. It is involved in the activity of insulin, in glucose tolerance in diabetes and in immune system function. It is also essential for the correct functioning of the voluntary muscles that move the bones and joints. Chromium is found in whole and unrefined foods, including wholemeal flour, whole grains, cereals, brewer's yeast, nuts, meat, liver, kidney and fresh fruits. A deficiency may cause irritability and depression, forgetfulness and sleep disturbances. The RDA is 0.05 to 0.2 mg.

Sulphur

Sulphur is involved in amino acid metabolism and the manufacture of proteins and hence it is important in the structural components of the body – bones, nails, teeth and skin. Sulphur-containing amino acids called methionine and cysteine are possibly involved in human longevity and tend to decline in older age. Good dietary sources of sulphur are eggs, meat, liver, pulses, garlic, onions, nuts, brewer's yeast, fish and dairy products. Deficiency is not reported and there is no RDA.

Strontium

Strontium is similar in composition to calcium and, like that mineral, is naturally found concentrated in bones and teeth. Strontium is obtained from foods such as milk and other dairy produce and helps to ensure the strength of bone and can be beneficial in the treatment of osteoporosis. The RDA is not known.

Boron

Boron is thought to be involved, as a trace element, in the utilisation of calcium and in the activity of vitamin D and the hormone oestrogen. Boron is found especially in fresh vegetables and fruits and can be beneficial in the treatment of osteoporosis. There is no RDA.

Free radicals and antioxidants

Free radicals are naturally-occurring, unstable compounds that are highly reactive. Their molecular structure enables them to freely attach to, and destroy, useful substances in the body thereby causing harm. The majority of free radicals are produced within the body but external sources include tobacco smoke, chemicals, exhaust emissions, radiation and alcohol. Substances that are able to counteract their activity and prevent damage are called antioxidants.

The body produces several antioxidant enzymes but some vitamins and minerals (e.g. vitamins C and E, selenium and sulphur) also have antioxidant activity. In addition, two groups of plant substances have been found to be very important and these are carotenes and flavonoids. Carotenes are molecules that contain carotenoids – orange, yellow or red pigments that are found quite widely in plants and in some animal tissues (egg yolk, milk, fat). Carotenes have potent antioxidant activity and it is believed that a high concentration within the body boosts immune system function and fights the free radical damage which is thought to be a significant factor in ageing. The best sources of carotenes are carrots, green, leafy vegetables, beets, sweet potatoes and many other vegetables.

Flavonoids are a group of naturally-occurring plant pigments that are widely found in fruits, particularly berries (e.g. blackberries, blackcurrants, cherries, bilberries, etc.) and in vegetables and flowers. In addition to having antioxidant activity and the ability to 'mop up' free radicals, they also appear to have anti-viral, anti-allergy, anti-inflammatory and anti-carcinogenic properties. A good intake of flavonoids can be ensured by eating a diet rich in fruit and vegetables.

Water
The human body is largely composed of water (66 per cent) which is essential to all life processes. Health experts recommend that eight glasses of, preferably, plain water should be drunk each day as a minimum amount. This factor is frequently overlooked by people who are dieting and it is thought that mild dehydration, which is not good for the body, is a fairly common occurrence. It is interesting to note that the first 'weight' which is lost by someone embarking on a reduced calorie diet is water!

Summary
It can be seen from the discussion above that human beings have complex nutritional needs and that food is not only needed for daily life but has an important protective role in preventing disease and prolonging longevity. In addition, convincing evidence is beginning to emerge of the importance of diet in fighting disease, if it does arise. Hence an understanding of basic nutrition is important for everyone but is particularly relevant for someone contemplating going on a diet. Some weight-loss plans and diets are quite restrictive and clearly do not fulfil the basic requirements of nutrition. The same may easily apply to people who are following their own individual, calorie-cutting programme on a fairly haphazard basis. A good example of this is the widely perceived view that foods such as potatoes and bread are fattening, with many dieters giving these up altogether. In fact, potatoes (especially with their skins) and bread (particularly wholemeal), are an excellent source of the most useful form of carbohydrate (starch) and of fibre, vitamins and minerals. Some of the problems associated with following a restricted diet can be avoided by taking a multivitamin/mineral supplement and by only staying on the plan for a certain period of time to achieve a specific weight loss. The most helpful restricted diet plans are those which give advice about returning to healthy, normal eating.

Why is Obesity a Problem for People in Western Countries?

STUDIES have shown that people in Britain, the USA and other western countries now run a greater risk of being overweight or obese than at almost any period in the past. Better nutrition in the years since the Second World War has led to people becoming larger and heavier than their forebears and, in women, there has been a change in basic body shape. A higher standard of nutrition is a positive development and should not, in itself, have caused the risk in the incidence of obesity. Health experts have identified two major factors which, working together, are held to be largely responsible: diet and lifestyle.

Diet and lifestyle

The first is, of course, related to the nature of the foods eaten. During the last half century, food has become increasingly refined and processed with a huge expansion in the number of 'convenience' foods available. Most of these foods are laden with hidden fats and sugar and bear little resemblance to their original raw materials. Coinciding with this, the pace of life has undoubtedly quickened beyond recognition.

In most modern households, there is no-one at home during the day – adults are at work and children at school. On returning home, sometimes quite late in the evening, people may feel too tired or otherwise disinclined to prepare and cook a meal so convenience food is chosen, which is ready in minutes when placed in a microwave oven. Often adults and children eat at different times and there is no opportunity to prepare and eat a family meal except at the weekend.

Most middle-aged people in Britain will probably be able to remember a very different pattern of eating from their own childhood. Then it was usual for meals to be prepared from raw ingredients on a daily basis and for a family to sit down and eat their dinner together. Through observation, children knew and understood the connection between the food on their plate and the raw ingredients from which it came. Foods were eaten in season so that the advent of particular vegetables and fruits was something which was eagerly anticipated – strawberries and other soft fruits in summer being a good example. Surveys have shown that modern children often have little idea about the origins of the food that they eat and do not realize how much it has been altered during processing. If very little cookery is taking place at home, children do not have the opportunity to naturally acquire knowledge about the way in which meals are made from raw ingredients. As noted above, ready-made meals tend to be high in fat and sugar although there are also low fat varieties available. However, the problem with all manufactured meals is that they lose a great many of their natural nutrients, particularly vitamins, during processing and rely heavily upon the addition of artificial chemical flavourings and colourings.

All this contrasts greatly with the opinion of nutritional experts who advise that food should be eaten in as natural a state as possible. People who follow this healthy pattern of eating obtain the full nutritional value from their food and are less likely to gain weight. This is because natural wholefoods are more satisfying and so less tends to be eaten, there are no 'hidden' calories and it is easily possible to adjust the diet to aid weight loss, if required.

Processed foods

The expansion in manufactured and processed foods has included an enormous rise in the availability and variety of snacks which are, of course, designed to be eaten between meals. Almost without exception, these foods are high in calories in the form of fat and sugar and people in Britain and other western countries eat them in huge quantities! It is thought that consumption of snacks or 'junk' foods, so-called because they provide little of use in the way of nutrition other than calories, contributes greatly to the problem of obesity. These foods are easy to eat and tend not to produce a feeling of fullness. They easily add many extra calories to the diet, almost without it being noticed – calories which are readily stored by the body as fat. In addition, snacks are often eaten while watching television or socialising with friends and studies suggest that people are far less aware of how much they are consuming under these circumstances.

Alcohol

Finally, drinking alcohol undoubtedly contributes towards weight gain and obesity in some adults and this may be a particular problem for men.

Like snacks, alcoholic drinks tend to be high in calories but contribute little else of nutritional value. Drinking oils the wheels of many of the social activities in which adults are engaged and sensible consumption of alcohol can be beneficial. There is little doubt, however, that alcohol is a hidden extra source of calories and one which is often not taken into account. Drinking is often accompanied by eating high calorie snack foods and so it can be appreciated just how easily a few evenings of socialising can add to the overall risk of weight gain.

Sedentary lifestyles

Even though the western diet has been shown to be unhealthy, particularly because of its high fat content, it appears that this alone cannot account for the epidemic in obesity. Traditional fare, both in Scotland and England, often included a daily fried breakfast, plenty of butter, full-fat dairy produce and fatty meats which would be considered unhealthy by modern standards, yet people were not as fat in the past as they are today.

The second major change which has taken place in the last 50 years and which is held to be accountable is in lifestyle. In the immediate post-war years, many more people were engaged in work which involved hard physical labour than is the case today. Also, few people owned cars so getting to work usually involved walking to catch buses or trains each day. Children walked to school and played outside and there were fewer labour-saving devices for the home so housework and gardening involved much harder physical work and greater expenditure of energy.

Without televisions and computers to keep leisure hours occupied, people were generally more active and the changes which have taken place are, in fact, quite profound. Most people in modern Britain have access to a wide range of labour-saving devices and technology which reduce the amount of physical effort needed for daily life.

The list of these seems almost endless and there is no doubt that such innovations have brought enormous benefits with new products appearing on the market all the time. Added to this is the fact that most households include at least one, if not two cars, and where people would once have walked, they now drive. To occupy their leisure hours, most families own one or several television sets (operated by remote control!) and computers. Even answering the telephone can now be carried out from an armchair!

Coinciding with these developments, and particularly affecting children, has been a change in the perceived dangers associated with the environment. Busy roads mean that few children are now allowed to walk to school and parental fear of 'stranger danger' means that they are not permitted to play outside. Perhaps not surprisingly, surveys have revealed that many children spend an enormous amount of their leisure time sitting in front of television and computer screens. Likewise, adults in Britain are often working long hours but most are engaged in sedentary occupations that require little physical expenditure of energy. The advent of new technology was expected to result in shorter working hours and more leisure time for people to pursue hobbies and sports. The reality is that many people are so busy that they find it difficult to make time for exercise while gadgets in the home allow us to be more idle than at any time in the past.

There is no doubt that physical activity helps to maintain a healthy weight and lessens the risk of obesity but the relationship between exercise and weight is a complex one which is discussed in more detail on page 70. What is certain is that people who live in societies where hard physical work has to be carried out just to obtain food and to sustain life on a daily basis are very seldom overweight or obese. However, it has been shown that if such people move to a western country and adopt a western diet and lifestyle, then their risk of obesity and associated illness, increases.

The most important aspect for any individual wishing to lose weight is to appreciate the impact that lifestyle may be having and to look at ways in which increased physical activity can be worked into the daily routine.

Health, Social and Psychological Problems of Obesity

BEING considerably overweight or obese carries with it a number of serious health risks which increase with age. These include elevated levels of cholesterol in the blood and atherosclerosis (narrowing of the arteries), heart and circulatory disease, stroke, hypertension (high blood pressure), diabetes, certain types of cancer and gall bladder disease. In addition, those who are overweight or obese are more likely to suffer from gout and arthritic conditions of the joints, especially affecting the hips and the knees. Physical exertion is more difficult and tiring for those who are overweight and these people may find that they lack energy. (An enhanced feeling of energy and enthusiasm for life is often reported by people who were formerly obese but who have lost their excess weight). A further, minor problem can be soreness and sweating where skin folds rub together. The occurrence of some of the conditions listed above can be life threatening and it is also a fact that obesity is linked to a shorter than expected lifespan.

Fat children

One worrying development is that evidence of furring of the arteries is increasingly being detected in today's children, who tend to be overweight and unfit. It is feared that these children are at risk of contracting, for example, heart and circulatory disease during young adult life, with all the possible consequences that this entails.

The social aspects of obesity can be quite profound, both for children and for adults. Fat children often suffer unkind teasing and/or bullying at school, as obesity makes a child an obvious target and many suffer great unhappiness as a result. A fat child may always feel on the outside of the peer group, may dread school sports lessons and often lacks self-confidence. Surveys have shown that children are acutely aware of the pressure exerted by the media and fashion industry, to be slim and that this awareness is dawning at an ever younger age. As a result, many children, particularly girls, who are of a normal size and weight believe that they are too fat and are unhappy with their body shape. It can be appreciated that if this is a common feeling among slim children then the pressure on those who are obese can be intense and considerable unhappiness can be the result. It is particularly unfortunate when it is realized that being chubby or having a covering of what used to be termed 'puppy fat' is perfectly normal during childhood but can still be the focus of teasing.

Even if a child is clearly overweight or obese, health experts agree that no-one under the age of 18 should embark upon a reducing diet, except under medical advice.

Instead the child should be encouraged to eat and above all enjoy a healthy, balanced diet which may mean that the whole family has to get involved and alter their eating habits.

Foods that are clearly fattening should not be banned but eaten infrequently as treats. Also, the child should be encouraged to take more exercise and this very often means finding an activity which the whole family can enjoy taking part in together. In the great majority of cases, fat children who eat healthily and take more exercise soon begin to lose their excess weight. This takes place naturally, without the child feeling hungry or deprived and, of course, once the process begins, there is a great incentive to continue. Very often, the whole family benefits too!

The key to success is thought to be fairly simple and not surprisingly, hinges upon parental support and encouragement. First and foremost, a parent should never comment negatively upon a child's weight or appearance. If the child really is fat and is unhappy as a result, then he or she will probably be receptive towards making the type of changes outlined above and will be pleased to be involved in the discussion. It may be appropriate to consult the family doctor if the child is willing to do so.

If parents are concerned that their child is too fat but the child himself has not noticed and is unconcerned, then it may be best to try and introduce changes more subtly, without comment. If and when the child notices that these are taking place, it can be explained that a more healthy eating pattern was felt to be better for the whole family. The older the child is, the more difficult it may become and teenagers, as every parent knows, have to be handled extremely carefully as they can be very sensitive to anything that sounds like criticism. The greatest risk for this age group is posed by eating disorders which, sadly, are becoming every more prevalent, At the end of the day, it is much better to have a non-dieting, junk-food eating, overweight but psychologically healthy child, who may decide later to change his or her eating habits, than one who, for whatever reason, embarks upon the destructive cycle of crash dieting or eating disorder.

A regime which is popular in America and was recently tried for the first time in Britain is that of the so-called 'Fat Camps' – summer camps for obese children. These camps are based upon a plan of healthy eating, combined with exercise and activities designed to appeal to children but aimed at achieving a loss in weight. Some people believe that it is wrong to single out children in this way. Others maintain that since all share the same problem it is, in fact, an easier environment for children who can take part in activities, perhaps for the first time, without fear of being singled out. It seems likely that the scheme will remain of minority interest in Britain which does not have the same tradition of children's summer camps as North America.

Social consequences for overweight people

The social consequences of being overweight or obese can be as severe for adults as they are for children and adults may be equally ill-equipped to deal with them. It is particularly unfortunate when overweight people, who may themselves be perfectly comfortable with their size, are made to feel unhappy or inferior by the insulting remarks of others.

It is not unusual for an overweight person to be on the receiving end of unkind and hurtful remarks from complete strangers, who are rude enough to believe that they have the right to comment on another person's appearance.

It is even worse when, as may sometimes happen, the remarks are made by a family member or friend. Derogatory remarks made on the grounds of race, colour, creed or disability rightly cause outrage in Britain and may even result in court action. Many believe that the same consideration should be afforded to fat (or thin) people as well although, of course, it is a difficult area for legislation.

Certainly, attitudes are not helped by the cultural and fashionable adulation of thinness that prevails in society. The 'thin is beautiful' viewpoint fosters the attitude held by some people that those who are overweight cannot, by definition, be physically attractive to others. Even more outrageous is the view that overweight people are less intelligent and somehow undeserving of society's approval. There is not a shred of evidence for any of these views but they are insidious and pervasive and so heavier people suffer as a result.

Discrimination

One of the manifestations of these views is that those who are obese far more commonly suffer discrimination in the workplace, being less likely to be successful at interviews for jobs or selected for promoted positions. Obviously, if this is occurring on a regular basis, and studies suggest that it is, then being fat can have serious financial consequences. Also, other surveys suggest that those who are overweight are more likely to be discriminated against in public places and on public transport and may not have their views taken seriously.

Overweight people have frequently found it difficult to buy fashionable and attractive clothes suitable for their size, although some manufacturers are now beginning to realize the marketing advantages of stocking larger sizes. There is evidence that the tide may finally be turning towards a more sensible attitude to the whole area of weight and the issues that surround it. This has partly been brought about by alarm over the increasing incidence of eating disorders among young women, especially with the fashion industry and media finally being held accountable for the harm caused by the image that they promote.

Big is beautiful

However, there has been a backlash from larger people themselves, including several of high profile, celebrity status whose views are not so easily dismissed, directed against the attitudes expressed by the fashion industry, media and tabloid newspapers. These people are proud to assert that they are happy and comfortable with their size, have no problem in attracting partners and, most importantly, that their appearance is nobody's business but their own. By publicising these hitherto unfashionable views, they have boosted the self-confidence of many ordinary, overweight people.

The fact remains that most larger people do not have difficulty in enjoying an active social life or finding a partner. In spite of the fashion industry and the media, surveys reveal that many ordinary people admire those of more ample proportions – Marilyn Monroe was a very curvaceous size 16! In addition, many find it repugnant when people are criticised by the media because of their size. One of the most distasteful examples in recent years was the lampooning of the Duchess of York, just days after she had given birth, which was justly condemned by medical experts. Those who dish out this kind of damaging criticism would do well to remember that they are far from perfect themselves!

Body image and self image

It is always worth bearing in mind that while being obese or very overweight is definitely bad for your health, being slightly, or even moderately overweight, is not. Hence, for many people the decision to diet is definitely a matter of choice rather than necessity and having a covering of fat (which is built into the genetic design of human beings), confers some advantages. For example, those who have body fat are able to survive longer when food is scarce or conditions are harsh as they are better able to withstand the cold. The female body needs fat in order to conceive and bear children.

Being slightly overweight has no effect on longevity; people in this situation can expect to enjoy as long a lifespan as they would do if they were slim. Perhaps one of the main disadvantages is that those who are already slightly overweight have fewer pounds to gain before they become obese and hence may wish to be careful about their diet.

The psychological consequences of being overweight or obese very much depend upon the nature of the individual concerned. Studies have shown that some large people are very unhappy about their size and suffer considerably as a result, often having low self-esteem and being locked into a cycle of dieting, frequently with little success. However, surveys reveal that people of slimmer proportions, especially young women, tend to be equally unhappy with their body shape and size. It seems that being comfortable with oneself can be an elusive commodity.

As mentioned on page 42, other large people are unconcerned and content to be the way they are and this viewpoint may be becoming more prevalent. It is far too easy for excess weight to become the sole focus of all personal unhappiness and dissatisfaction – a peg on which to hang all life's woes. Someone in this position does not necessarily achieve happiness after successful dieting but may discover other problems which had previously been masked.

Others, however, have found that a new, more confident and happy self emerged as a result of a loss in weight. So much depends upon individual temperament, but it serves to highlight the fact that an honest appraisal of personal aspirations and motives is a worthwhile exercise for any would-be dieter. The role of self-evaluation is discussed in more detail on page 77 (see Points to Consider).

The Mechanisms of
Hunger and Appetite

MOST people probably feel from their own experience that they understand the meaning of hunger and appetite. References to someone being 'always hungry', having 'a good appetite' or having 'lost his appetite' are often used and readily understood. It is, however, useful to examine these two factors a little more closely and in particular to see if there are any differences in the experience of them between those who are fat and those who are slim. Hunger is the sensation of needing food in order to provide the body with the substances it needs to perform bodily functions. The sensation of hunger is believed to arise as a result of the contractions of an empty stomach but this, in itself is mediated by complex biochemical processes interpreted by the brain. The mechanism is a complicated one which remains imperfectly understood. Appetite is the desire to eat food and again, it is ultimately controlled by the brain, interpreting signals both from within and outside the body. Also, it has been discovered that the operation of a good or a poor appetite depends upon the muscular tone of the stomach. Once again, the mechanisms at work in the operation of appetite are not entirely understood. Appetite and hunger are evidently closely linked but it seems that the factors affecting appetite are mostly learned and acquired. This is supported by the fact that the appetite can be stimulated by the sight and smell of delicious food, so that a person may then eat even though not hungry. Conversely, the sight or smell or something revolting, that is not necessarily food, can take away the appetite and the desire to eat, even though the person may, in fact, be hungry.

Illness can depress both appetite and hunger and people may find it difficult to eat enough to aid recovery. Also, some conditions and disorders can cause the appetite to go awry or become depraved. Pregnancy and the development of cravings for certain, often unusual, foods is one example and pica, an abnormal desire to eat inappropriate substances such as soap, chalk, soil, etc., which sometimes affects children, is another.

In theory, people should be able to 'eat for need, not greed' and just consume enough food to satisfy hunger, stopping when they feel full. However, studies show that the experience of feeling hungry and feeling full varies greatly between different people and that it takes more food to satisfy some than others. Studies have been carried out to try an discover if fatter people are less readily satisfied than thinner ones, i.e. whether the 'feeling full' signal operates poorly so that they eat more. However, no significant differences have been found between the two groups. Also, as indicated above, stimulation of the appetite can make someone feel hungry, whether they actually need to eat or not. As has been seen, the gaining of weight (or not), then depends upon the nature of the food eaten, lifestyle and certain physical factors which are discussed in more detail below.

Appetite and hunger are ultimately under the control of the brain but the way in which regulatory mechanisms operate is not fully understood. Further elucidation of these mechanisms may, in the future, be helpful in the prevention of obesity.

Psychological aspects of food and eating

Most people would probably be readily able to accept that, at least for some of the time, they do not eat merely to satisfy hunger. Mention has been made on page 44 of the powerful effect of having the appetite stimulated by the sight and smell of delicious food – a factor which is exploited by supermarkets that use the aroma of baking bread to attract customers to their bakery shelves! There can be very few people who have not succumbed to the temptation to eat something which looks or tastes inviting, or is perhaps an unusual new food which they have not tried before. Food manufacturers employ many strategies to try to persuade consumers to buy their products and people in western countries are bombarded with new foods and drinks which appear on the market almost on a daily basis. As already stated, many of these foods are of a type that is high in calories. Advertising, special offers such as money-off coupons or 'buy one get one free' and placing tempting products at the checkout counter are used relentlessly. Hence it is hardly surprising that people may return home with products that they did not intend to buy and that the whole business of food marketing contributes to the problem of obesity.

If food manufacturers and supermarkets exploit two main aspects of human psychology to tempt their customers to buy – that of greed and people's love of a bargain – these are not the only factors at work in determining patterns of eating. In every human society, food forms an immensely important part of social and cultural inter-relationships. Food is used to signal friendship, hospitality and love and, all over the world, holidays are feast days. The great events in family (and national) life are virtually always celebrated by people serving the best food that they can manage to produce. Hence the rejection of food can be a cause of great offence and has even been given as a reason for the outbreaks of feuds and fighting. Likewise, the withholding or denial of food – for example from a child – is a sign of disapproval and displeasure just as rewards, in the form of edible treats, signal approval and affection. Western peoples are imbued with these social and cultural aspects of food from an early age. Probably every reader will have had the experience of visiting a relative or friend who has produced a plateful of home-made cakes, along with the tea or coffee, and who would have felt hurt if their visitor had not eaten one. This is often cited by the clergy as one of the occupational hazards (to their waistlines) of their calling! On being invited out to dinner, most people would try to eat the meal which is produced, even if it is something which they normally do not like, rather than risk causing hurt or offence by refusing.

In Britain, almost all elderly people have had direct experience of food shortages, rationing and deprivation during the years of the Second World War. Hence their children, those who are now middle-aged, were commonly brought up to unquestioningly eat every morsel of food that someone else had placed on their plate and were punished (at school if not at home) if they did not do so. This type of training is hard to shake off and although subsequent generations of children have generally experienced a more relaxed attitude to eating, it is still difficult for many people to leave or waste food. From all the above, it can be readily appreciated that for western people, there is a great deal more involved in eating food than the mere satisfaction of hunger.

The social side of food is often a difficult area for people trying to lose weight as they can easily be made to feel that they are spoiling the party! Very often, people are urged either to forget their diet for that one occasion or, faced with an array of appetising, diet-breaking foods, find themselves unable to resist the temptation to eat. Strategies for keeping to your diet plan on social occasions, without falling out with your friends, are outlined in a later section! Another psychological factor which influences eating, at least in some people for part of the time, is their emotional state. When unhappy, some people turn to food for comfort, often eating unsuitable items which are high in fat and sugar such as biscuits or chocolate. Likewise, when worried or distressed, some people eat more, others find it difficult to eat at all, while some are unaffected. Worry is, in fact, one aspect of stress – a state which causes physiological changes in the body which themselves affect the appetite. The reasons behind 'comfort eating' are complex and may be a reflection of deep-rooted unhappiness or insecurity or other factors which are difficult for the person to identify. In other cases, the person may be aware of the problem and that he or she is eating to compensate for some difficult problem in life. However, not surprisingly, those who regularly comfort eat are at a higher risk of gaining excess weight and becoming obese. Probably the best solution for a comfort eater is to try to identify the cause of the problem, perhaps with the help of a sympathetic family member, close friend or GP. Even the most intractable of problems can often be lessened by sharing it with somebody else and sometimes all that is needed is a little positive support and help.

Cravings for a variety of foods which are not associated with any particular disorder or condition, are another common experience that appears to have an entirely psychological basis. Although cravings are often short term, 'one-off', infrequent occurrences that disappear once the particular, desired food is eaten, they may sometimes persist for longer and do play a part in determining what people eat. Perhaps not surprisingly, it is often in conditions of deprivation (including that imposed by a strict diet) when people experience the strongest cravings for unobtainable or 'forbidden' foods that they have previously enjoyed. Cravings can involve any kind of food but those on a diet often feel a longing for something that is rich, fattening and unsuitable! These feelings can be particularly strong in the early days of a diet before the person has had time to adapt to the new regime of eating. As far as the problem of weight gain and obesity is concerned, they are probably of minor significance. Cravings can, nonetheless, be the bane of a dieter since they can be difficult to banish from the mind. Three solutions are possible. The first is to occupy oneself with an enjoyable alternative activity which will hopefully divert attention away from the cravings. The second is to eat a low calorie equivalent of the food that one craves, if one exists and this is a realistic possibility. The third is to succumb to the craving on this one occasion and eat and enjoy a portion of the food, while resolving not to have it again for at least another week, or longer!

Eating Disorders

THE most serious psychological conditions connected with food and eating in the western world are the eating disorders anorexia nervosa and bulimia nervosa. Both of these are highly complex conditions which, although centred around food, are in fact manifestations of severe psychological disturbance and distress. Both conditions have become ever more prevalent in recent years, affecting mainly teenagers and young adults and especially girls and young women. Of great concern is the fact that eating disorders are increasingly being reported in children from the age of about 11 years upwards and are not unknown in even younger children. In May 2000, the British Medical Association published a report entitled *Eating Disorders, Body Image and the Media*. The report laid much of the blame for the inexorable rise in these conditions at the door of the fashion and media industries for perpetuating an unhealthy image of thinness, equated with beauty, which is unobtainable for most young women. The fashion industry has hit back by saying that they are now, in fact, using larger models but that in any event, they are only responding to public demand by promoting thinness. Both of these arguments have a very hollow ring to them. Research has shown that the average successful model or actress has only 10 to 15 per cent body fat compared to 22 to 26 per cent for a normal, healthy woman. In order to try to succeed in the world of fashion and media, or to emulate those that do, many young women are going without food and all this at a time when the average size for British women has increased from a 12 to a 14. Also, as discussed previously, it is not the case that ordinary people universally find extreme thinness to be attractive. Surveys consistently reveal that most would prefer to see images of attractive people of average size promoted by the media and that there is a great deal of concern about the rise in incidence of eating disorders.

The power of the media in influencing people's ideas about themselves has been demonstrated by the advent of western television broadcasting to Fiji in 1995. Since western programmes have been shown, there has been an explosion in dieting among Fijian teenagers who were previously not concerned about their weight. In Britain, eating disorders continue to exact their toll of suffering upon victims and their families, with both well known and ordinary people being affected. In Scotland, there are at least 6000 people suffering from an eating disorder at any particular time and 90 per cent of these are young women. Up to 20 per cent of them die within 20 years from the physical effects of their disorder and even those who survive and are cured can suffer permanent bodily damage.

Anorexia nervosa

Anorexia nervosa is a psychological disorder in which the victim, who is usually young and female, avoids food and starves herself to such an extent that there is a severe and dangerous loss of weight. Its characteristic feature is that the victim has a false and distorted image of herself as being obese, so that when she looks in the mirror she sees a fat person. This generates feelings of disgust and self-loathing and a fear of obesity, amounting to phobia, which renders the victim unable to eat normally. Anorexics are often beset by feelings of shame and secrecy and go to great lengths to conceal their abnormal eating habits and loss of weight from friends and family. If challenged, they deny feeling hunger or that they have a problem and can become quite angry. Self-starvation can be accompanied by excessive exercise, use of laxatives and self-induced vomiting to further promote weight loss. As the weight plummets, menstruation stops, blood pressure falls, there may be vitamin and mineral deficiencies and anaemia, and growth of lanugo – a downy, body hair which the body produces in an attempt to conserve heat and energy. Eventually, body tissues and organs begin to be broken down and there is a serious risk of permanent damage to the heart and sudden death from heart attack. Anorexics commonly suffer from severe depression, some to the point of suicide.

The reasons behind anorexia are complex and while incidence has increased in recent years, evidence suggests that it is a condition which has occasionally arisen throughout history. There is undoubtedly a link with the fashionable and cultural ideal of thinness but it is thought that those who become anorexic are vulnerable in other ways as well. Anorexia commonly develops during adolescence or in the teenage years, at a time when the child is becoming an adult, new feelings and ideas are being experienced and family relationships may be changing. Experts believe that all these factors may be relevant and that anorexia is a reflection of deep psychological insecurity. By denying herself food, the young person may be attempting to somehow reassert control over her life or reverse the process of becoming a sexually functioning adult. Anorexia may also be triggered by profound emotional changes accompanying, for example, separation of parents, bereavement and grief or leaving home.

Whatever the cause, anorexics require specialist help although treatment of the condition can be a prolonged and difficult matter. Specialist residential care and psychotherapy are generally the most successful options but where life is threatened, hospitalization and force feeding may be the only option. Anyone who suspects that a child or friend has anorexia should seek professional help by initially alerting the family doctor, even if the victim herself is uncooperative. Professional support groups exist to help both the victim and her family and the sooner discussion and therapy begin, the sooner progress can be made towards recovery.

Bulimia nervosa

Bulimia nervosa is characterised by binge eating, followed by induced vomiting and misuse of laxatives to avoid any gain in weight. Once again, the victim is usually a young woman who believes that she is at risk of obesity and develops a fear of food. Yet she experiences craving for food and binges in order to satisfy herself. The victim is often full of self-disgust, has low self-esteem and tries to conceal her eating habits from others. Bulimia may result in vitamin and mineral deficiencies, gastric problems and ulcers, rotting of teeth and mouth ulcers (caused by stomach acid entering the mouth during frequent vomiting), swelling of joints and disruption of the menstrual cycle. Most bulimics are able to function normally and maintain a reasonable weight, but in severe and persistent cases, there is a risk of kidney damage, low blood pressure, circulatory problems and dehydration. Bulimia is often accompanied by unhappiness and depression and experts believe that in vulnerable people, it may be triggered by dieting. As with anorexia, it is thought that one of the causes of bulimia is the pressure felt by young people to be thin. The abnormal pattern of eating and purging may arise out of dissatisfaction or hatred of one's body shape and size but may also be a reflection of deeper problems and unhappiness. Anyone who suspects that a family member or friend is suffering from bulimia should try to engage in a sympathetic discussion of the problem and offer support. If the person is cooperative, professional help can be sought through the family doctor which may involve psychotherapy, counselling and possible use of antidepressants. Also, there are support groups which can provide a great deal of help for individual sufferers and their families.

Anorexia and bulimia are distressing and damaging disorders but in many cases they can be cured.

The address of the Eating Disorders Association is given on page 287.

Binge eating

A third type of eating disorder affecting obese persons has recently been defined. This is called binge eating disorder and it affects older adults of both sexes in equal numbers. It is characterized by binge eating, but without subsequent misuse of laxatives or induced vomiting and so it may be largely responsible for a person's obesity and lack of success in dieting. People suffering from this disorder are often trying to lose weight and are distressed that their lack of control over binge eating which is hindering their efforts to do so. Psychotherapy and the use of appetite suppressant drugs and possibly anti-depressants can help. However, many people remain untreated since the primary problem is seen to be their obesity and they may not admit to a disordered pattern of eating. Psychotherapy, along with dietary advice so that the person begins to achieve the desired reduction in weight, seems to offer the best chance of a cure.

Physical Aspects of Obesity –
The Role of Genes

FOR many years, there has been considerable debate, both in public and scientific circles, about the exact nature and causes of obesity. In simple terms, there are two basic schools of thought, the first and most obvious one being that obesity is always the result of over-indulgence. This attitude is easily understood and highly entrenched in western society. Most people believe that an overweight or fat person has become that way through simply eating too much and hence the remedy is to reduce the amount or type of food consumed.

However, there is a second school of thought, and one which forms an area of scientific research, which holds that a tendency for obesity is determined by inherited genetic factors. It is obvious that genes determine the basic provision and distribution of fat in the human species and that these factors once conferred an evolutionary advantage.

As previously stated, humans are naturally fat compared to many other mammals and the ability to store fat is advantageous in times of food shortage. Also, women need fat in order to successfully reproduce and menstruation fails if their reserves are depleted below the critical level of 17 per cent of body weight as fat. In addition, genetic differences between the various races of people may play some part in determining the likelihood of obesity.

Metabolism
However, the most critical role played by genes is believed to be through their control of metabolism. This is the sum of all the physical and chemical changes within cells and tissues which are necessary for life and which are fuelled by the energy derived from food. Basal metabolism is the amount of energy required to maintain the body's vital processes, such as heartbeat, respiration and maintenance of body temperature, while the body is at rest and this varies between different people. In theory, if a person's metabolic requirements are high, the greater the likelihood that calories from food will be utilised to provide energy rather than being laid down as fat. Basal

metabolic rate is higher in children and young adults than in older people. Muscle requires more energy than fat, and since males have more muscle and less fat compared to females, their basal metabolic rate is generally higher although this varies considerably between individuals. The significance of differences in metabolism between individual people in controlling obesity is the subject of debate. However, it certainly seems to be true that some people are able to eat more or less what they like without gaining weight – and most dieters know at least one of them!

Conversely, others may have to constantly watch what they eat in order to maintain a reasonable weight and find that any lapses or indulgences are noticed when they next stand on the bathroom scales! Scientists working at the universities of Edinburgh and Aberdeen have been conducting research into the genetic control of metabolism, looking for a so-called anti-obesity gene. They recently announced that they have developed a strain of mice that are able to eat 40 per cent more food than ordinary mice without gaining weight. It is thought that these slim but greedy mice possess one or more genes that ensure that their metabolism uses up the calories from food rather than laying them down as fat. It is believed that this is achieved by more of the calories from food being converted into heat. This thermic effect of eating is a natural process which also occurs when humans consume food. In the next few years, it is hoped that the relevant genes will be isolated in both mice and humans and that a means of activating them can be found which should prove useful in the treatment and prevention of obesity. However, other experts continue to sound a note of caution. They state the metabolism is only one of the factors at work in obesity and may not be the most important one. They believe that for most people, the answer to reducing weight lies in a change in eating habits and lifestyle. Even if an anti-obesity gene is eventually located and can be activated so that a person's metabolism utilises calories more effectively, a healthy diet and lifestyle will still be necessary to protect against the risk of heart disease and cancer.

In summary, it seems likely that individual genetic factors, including those affecting metabolism, do influence a person's susceptibility to gain weight and this is hardly surprising since genes determine all the physical characteristics of the body. However, for most people, factors within their own control – diet, lifestyle and exercise – will determine whether they gain weight, become obese or maintain their weight at a reasonable level.

Determining the Need to Diet

AS stated previously, it is only necessary to diet to safeguard your health if your weight is sufficiently great to put you at risk of developing the disorders of obesity such as high blood pressure, heart and circulatory disease and diabetes.

Body mass index (BMI)

In order to determine when this point is reached, scientists and doctors use a formula known as the body mass index, or BMI, which is calculated from measurements of height and weight. A scale of numbers is derived, ranging from 'morbidly obese' at the top to 'emaciated' at the bottom and each person is classified according to his or her individual reading. The BMI figure is arrived at by using the following calculation:

weight (in kilograms) ÷ height (in metres) squared i.e.

$$\frac{\text{weight in kg}}{\text{height in m}^2}$$

To derive your height in metres, calculate your height in inches and divide the number by 40, i.e.:

$$\frac{\text{height in inches}}{40}$$

To derive your weight in kilograms, calculate your weight in pounds and divide the number by 2.2, i.e.:

$$\frac{\text{weight in pounds}}{2.2}$$

Example

A woman 5 ft 4 in tall is 64/40 in = 1.6 metres high and weighing 9 stone 7 lbs (133lbs) is 133/2.2 = 60.45 kg.

Hence her BMI is:

$$\frac{60.45 \text{ kg}}{1.6\text{m}^2} = \frac{60.45}{1.6 \times 1.6} = \frac{60.45}{2.56} = 23.6$$

Since these calculations are quite complex BMIs for both metric and Imperial measurements are given in tables 1 and 2 on pages 55 to 60. Find your height and weight on one of the charts to discover your round BMI figure.

Table 1: BMI Imperial Measurements

Your height in inches

Weight in pounds

Weight	58	59	60	61	62	63	64	65	66	67	68	69	70	71	72
90	19	18	18	17	16	16	15	15	15	14	14	13	13	13	12
92	19	19	18	17	17	16	16	15	15	14	14	14	13	13	12
94	20	19	18	18	17	17	16	16	15	15	14	14	13	13	13
96	20	19	19	18	18	17	16	16	15	15	15	14	14	13	13
98	20	20	19	19	18	17	17	16	16	15	15	14	14	14	13
100	21	20	20	19	18	18	17	17	16	16	15	15	14	14	14
102	21	21	20	19	19	18	18	17	16	16	16	15	15	14	14
104	22	21	20	20	19	18	18	17	17	16	16	15	15	15	14
106	22	21	21	20	19	19	18	18	17	17	16	16	15	15	14
108	23	22	21	20	20	19	19	18	17	17	16	16	15	15	15
110	23	22	21	21	20	19	19	18	18	17	17	16	16	15	15
112	23	23	22	21	20	20	19	19	18	18	17	17	16	16	15
114	24	23	22	22	21	20	20	19	18	18	17	17	16	16	15
116	24	23	23	22	21	21	20	19	19	18	18	17	17	16	16
118	25	24	23	22	22	21	20	20	19	18	18	17	17	16	16
120	25	24	23	23	22	21	21	20	19	19	18	18	17	17	16
122	26	25	24	23	22	22	21	20	20	19	19	18	18	17	17
124	26	25	24	23	23	22	21	21	20	19	19	18	18	17	17
126	26	25	25	24	23	22	22	21	20	20	19	19	18	18	17
128	27	26	25	24	23	23	22	21	21	20	20	19	18	18	17

Your height in inches

Weight in pounds	58	59	60	61	62	63	64	65	66	67	68	69	70	71	72
130	27	26	25	25	24	23	22	22	21	20	20	19	19	18	18
132	28	27	26	25	24	23	23	22	21	21	20	20	19	18	18
134	28	27	26	25	25	24	23	22	22	21	20	20	19	19	18
136	29	28	27	26	25	24	23	23	22	21	21	20	20	19	18
138	29	28	27	26	25	25	24	23	22	22	21	20	20	19	19
140	29	28	27	27	26	25	24	23	23	22	21	21	20	19	19
142	30	29	28	27	26	25	25	24	23	22	22	21	20	20	19
144	30	29	28	27	26	26	25	24	23	23	22	21	21	20	20
146	31	30	29	28	27	26	25	24	24	23	22	22	21	20	20
148	31	30	29	28	27	26	26	25	24	23	23	22	21	21	20
150	31	30	29	28	28	27	26	25	24	24	23	22	22	21	20
152	32	31	30	29	28	27	26	26	25	24	23	23	22	21	21
154	32	31	30	29	28	27	27	26	25	24	24	23	22	22	21
156	33	32	31	30	29	28	27	26	26	25	24	23	23	22	21
158	33	32	31	30	29	28	27	26	26	25	24	24	23	22	22
160	34	32	31	30	29	28	28	27	26	25	25	24	23	23	22
162	34	33	32	31	30	29	28	27	26	26	25	24	24	23	22
164	34	33	32	31	30	29	28	27	27	26	25	25	24	23	23
166	35	34	33	32	31	30	29	28	27	26	25	25	24	23	23
168	35	34	33	32	31	30	29	28	27	26	26	25	24	24	23
170	36	34	33	32	31	30	29	28	28	27	26	25	24	24	23
172	36	35	34	33	32	31	30	29	28	27	26	25	25	24	23

174	176	178	180	182	184	186	188	190	192	194	196	198	200	202	204	206	208	210	212	214	216	218	220
24	24	24	24	25	25	25	26	26	26	26	27	27	27	27	28	28	28	29	29	29	29	30	30
24	25	25	25	25	26	26	26	27	27	27	27	28	28	28	29	29	29	29	30	30	30	30	31
25	25	26	26	26	26	27	27	27	28	28	28	28	29	29	29	30	30	30	31	31	31	31	32
26	26	26	27	27	27	28	28	28	28	29	29	29	30	30	30	31	31	31	31	32	32	32	33
27	27	27	27	28	28	28	29	29	29	30	30	30	30	31	31	31	32	32	32	33	33	33	34
27	28	28	28	29	29	29	30	30	30	31	31	31	32	32	32	33	33	33	34	34	34	34	35
28	28	29	29	29	30	30	30	31	31	31	32	32	32	33	33	33	34	34	34	35	35	35	36
29	29	29	30	30	30	31	31	31	32	32	32	33	33	33	34	34	34	35	35	35	36	36	37
30	30	31	31	31	31	32	32	32	33	33	33	34	34	34	35	35	35	36	36	36	37	37	38
31	31	32	32	32	33	33	33	34	34	34	35	35	36	36	36	37	37	37	38	38	39	39	39
32	32	33	33	33	34	34	34	35	35	36	36	36	37	37	37	38	38	39	39	39	40	40	40
33	33	34	34	34	35	35	36	36	36	37	37	38	38	38	39	39	39	40	40	41	41	41	42
34	34	35	35	36	36	36	37	37	38	38	38	39	39	40	40	40	41	41	42	42	42	43	43
35	36	36	36	37	37	38	38	38	39	39	40	40	41	41	41	42	42	43	43	43	44	44	45
36	37	37	38	38	39	39	39	40	40	41	41	41	42	42	43	43	44	44	44	45	45	46	46

Table 2: BMI Metric Measurements

Your height in centimetres

Weight in kg	150	152.5	155	157.5	160	162.5	165	167.5	170	172.5	175	177.5	180	182.5	185	187.5	190
40	18	17	17	16	16	15	15	14	14	13	13	13	12	12	12	11	11
41	18	18	17	17	16	16	15	15	14	14	13	13	13	12	12	12	11
42	19	18	17	17	16	16	15	15	15	14	14	13	13	13	12	12	12
43	19	18	18	17	17	16	16	15	15	14	14	14	13	13	13	12	12
44	20	19	18	18	17	17	16	16	15	15	14	14	14	13	13	13	12
45	20	19	19	18	18	17	17	16	16	15	15	14	14	14	13	13	13
46	20	20	19	19	18	17	17	16	16	15	15	15	14	14	13	13	13
47	21	20	20	19	18	18	17	17	16	16	15	15	14	14	14	13	13
48	21	21	20	19	19	18	18	17	17	16	16	15	15	14	14	14	13
49	22	21	20	20	19	19	18	17	17	16	16	16	15	15	14	14	14
50	22	21	21	20	20	19	18	18	17	17	16	16	15	15	15	14	14
51	23	22	21	21	20	19	19	18	18	17	17	16	16	15	15	14	14
52	23	22	22	21	20	20	19	18	18	17	17	17	16	16	15	15	14
53	24	23	22	21	21	20	19	19	18	18	17	17	16	16	15	15	15
54	24	23	22	22	21	20	20	19	19	18	18	17	17	16	16	15	15
55	24	24	23	22	21	21	20	20	19	18	18	17	17	17	16	16	15
56	25	24	23	23	22	21	21	20	19	19	18	18	17	17	16	16	16
57	25	25	24	23	22	22	21	20	20	19	18	18	18	17	17	16	16
58	26	25	24	23	23	22	21	21	20	19	19	18	18	17	17	16	16

59	16	17	17	18	18	19	19	20	20	21	22	22	23	24	25	25	26
60	17	17	18	18	19	19	20	20	21	21	22	23	23	24	25	26	27
61	17	17	18	18	19	19	20	20	21	22	22	23	24	25	25	26	27
62	17	18	18	19	19	20	20	21	21	22	23	23	24	25	26	27	28
63	17	18	18	19	19	20	21	21	22	22	23	24	25	25	26	27	28
64	18	18	19	19	20	20	21	22	22	23	24	24	25	26	27	28	28
65	18	18	19	20	20	21	21	22	22	23	24	25	25	26	27	28	29
66	18	19	19	20	21	21	22	22	23	24	24	25	26	27	27	28	29
67	19	19	20	20	21	21	22	23	23	24	25	25	26	27	28	29	30
68	19	19	20	21	21	22	22	23	24	24	25	26	27	27	28	29	30
69	19	20	20	21	22	22	23	23	24	25	25	26	27	28	29	30	31
70	19	20	21	21	22	22	23	24	24	25	26	26	27	28	29	30	31
71	20	20	21	22	22	23	23	24	25	25	26	27	28	29	30	31	32
72	20	21	21	22	23	23	24	24	25	26	26	27	28	29	30	31	32
73	20	21	22	23	23	23	24	25	25	26	27	27	29	29	30	31	32
74	20	21	22	23	23	24	24	25	26	26	27	28	29	30	31	32	33
75	21	22	22	23	24	24	24	25	26	27	28	28	29	30	31	32	33
76	21	22	23	23	24	24	25	25	26	27	28	28	30	31	32	33	34
77	21	22	23	24	24	25	25	26	27	27	28	29	30	31	32	33	34
78	22	23	23	24	25	25	26	26	27	28	29	29	30	31	32	34	35
79	22	23	24	24	25	25	26	27	27	28	29	30	31	32	33	34	35
80	22	23	24	25	25	26	26	27	28	29	29	30	31	32	33	34	36
81	22	23	24	25	26	26	27	27	28	29	30	31	32	33	34	35	36
82	23	23	24	25	26	26	27	28	28	29	30	31	32	33	34	35	36

Table 2: BMI Metric Measurements

Your height in centimetres

Weight in kg	150	152.5	155	157.5	160	162.5	165	167.5	170	172.5	175	177.5	180	182.5	185	187.5	190
83	37	36	35	33	32	31	30	30	29	28	27	26	26	25	24	24	23
84	37	36	35	34	33	32	31	30	29	28	27	27	26	25	25	24	23
85	38	37	35	34	33	32	31	30	29	29	28	27	26	26	25	24	24
86	38	37	36	35	34	33	32	31	30	29	28	27	27	26	25	24	24
87	39	37	36	35	34	33	32	31	30	29	28	28	27	26	25	25	24
88	39	38	37	35	34	33	32	31	30	30	29	28	27	26	26	25	24
89	40	38	37	36	35	34	33	32	31	30	29	28	27	27	26	25	25
90	40	39	37	36	35	34	33	32	31	30	29	29	28	27	26	25	25
91	40	39	38	37	36	34	33	32	31	31	30	29	28	27	27	26	25
92	41	40	38	37	36	35	34	33	32	31	30	29	28	28	27	26	25
93	41	40	39	37	36	35	34	33	32	31	30	30	29	28	27	26	26
94	42	40	39	38	37	36	35	34	33	32	31	30	29	28	27	27	26
95	42	41	40	39	37	36	35	34	33	32	31	30	29	29	28	27	26
96	43	41	40	39	38	36	35	34	33	32	31	30	30	29	28	27	27
97	43	42	40	39	38	37	36	35	34	33	32	31	30	29	28	28	27
98	44	42	41	40	38	37	36	35	34	33	32	31	30	29	28	28	27
99	44	43	41	40	39	37	36	35	34	33	32	31	31	30	29	28	27
100	44	43	42	40	39	38	37	36	35	34	33	32	31	30	29	28	28

The BMI scale is classified as follows:

Less than 15	Emaciated
15 to 19	Underweight
19 to 25	Average
25 to 27	Overweight
27 to 30	Overweight and at risk of developing obesity-related diseases
30 to 40	Obese and at high risk of disease
40 +	Morbidly obese

Designation of the optimum BMI range, associated with the lowest risk of weight-related conditions and illnesses, varies somewhat between different countries. However, in general terms, an optimum BMI for adults lies within the range of 20 to 25. For women it is in the order of 18.8 to 23.4 and for men, 19.8 to 24. Anyone lying slightly above or slightly below these figures is not at risk but still might wish to keep an eye on their weight. In fact using the example given above of a woman 5 ft 4 in tall; with an optimum BMI range of 20 to 25, her weight could be anything from 8 st 4 lbs (52.7 kg) to 10 st 8 lbs. (67 kg). In order to reach the danger zone of a BMI of 27, when she would be at risk of developing obesity-related diseases, her weight would need to climb to 11 st 3 lbs (71.3 kg) or above.

However, it is probable that at this weight, or even some way below it, many women would feel that they would like to lose a few pounds! Conversely, women especially, are at some risk if their BMI is too low and anyone with a figure of 19 or below should make sure that they are eating a full, healthy, well-balanced diet. No one with a BMI of less than 20 should go on a diet – with this reading, you cannot be overweight. Equally, if your BMI is 30 or above, seek medical advice about losing weight rather than embarking upon a diet on your own.

BMI is the most reliable measurement for determining health risks associated with weight but, as has been seen, it allows for considerable variation. Other figures that are used, especially by diet books and the diet industry in general, are so-called 'standard', 'average' or 'ideal' weight for height charts for men and women. These can be extremely variable, depending upon which book you are reading and should only be used as a rough guide. It is, after all, in the interests of the diet industry to promote ideal weights on the lower scale in order to recruit potential dieters! Weight charts are often based on ideal or standard weights for young adults and fail to take into account that people naturally tend to get a little heavier in middle and older age. Health experts advise people to try to retain the weight and clothes size that they had in youth (as long as they were not overweight). However, it may be more realistic to try and remain within sight of that weight and to keep muscles well-toned by taking plenty of exercise!

Frame size

The most useful weight charts are those which take into account body frame size, i.e. the mass of the internal skeleton. In general, women have a smaller body frame than men (although there is inevitably some overlap between the two) but people of the same sex and height also vary considerably in bone structure. A common excuse among those who are somewhat overweight is to assert that it is because they have 'large bones' but, in fact, the skeleton is relatively light compared to soft tissue! A large-framed person can expect to weigh more than one with a smaller frame and can more readily accommodate extra weight without appearing to be fat. Frame size can be estimated by measuring the width of the arm at the elbow. In order to do this, you should place a piece of paper on a table and then kneel or sit facing it and place your upper arm on the

Table 3: Medium frame determined by elbow width

WOMEN		MEN	
Height in m and feet	Elbow width in cm and ins	Height in m and feet	Elbow width in cm and ins
1.45 to 1.47 m	5.7 cm	1.55 to 1.60 m	6.4 to 7 cm
(4' 9" to 4' 10")	(2" to 2+")	(5' 1" to 5' 3")	(2+" to 2+")
1.50 to 1.57 m	5.4 to 6.4 cm	1.63 to 1.68 m	6.7 to 7.3 cm
(4' 11" to 5' 2")	(2" to 2+")	(5' 4" to 5' 6")	(2" to 2")
1.60 to 1.68 m	5.7 to 6.7 cm	1.70 to 1.78 m	7 to 7.6 cm
(5' 3" to 5' 6")	(2+" to 2")	(5' 7" to 5' 10")	(2+" to 3")
1.70 to 1.78 m	6 to 7 cm	1.80 to 1.88 m	7.3 to 7.9 cm
(5' 7" to 5' 10")	(2" to 2+")	(5'11" to 6' 2")	(2 " to 3")
1.80 to 1.85 m	6.4 to 7.3 cm	1.90 to 1.93 m	7.6 to 8.3 cm
(5'11" to 6'1")	(2+" to 3")	(6' 3" to 6' 4")	(3" to 3+")

Table 4: Tables for standard body weight

MEN

Height ft (m)	Small Frame lbs (kg)	Medium Frame lbs (kg)	Large Frame lbs (kg)
5' 1" (1.55)	107–130 (49–59)	113–134 (51–61)	121–140 (55–64)
5' 2" (1.57)	110–132 (50–60)	116–138 (53–63)	124–144 (56–65)
5' 3" (1.60)	113–134 (51–61)	119–140 (54–64)	127–150 (58–68)
5' 4" (1.63)	116–135 (53–61)	122–142 (55–65)	131–154 (59–70)
5' 5" (1.65)	119–137 (54–62)	125–146 (57–66)	133–159 (60–72)
5' 6" (1.68)	123–140 (56–64)	129–149 (59–68)	137–163 (62–74)
5' 7" (1.70)	127–143 (58–65)	133–152 (60–69)	142–167 (64–76)
5' 8" (1.73)	131–145 (60–66)	137–155 (62–71)	146–171 (66–78)
5' 9" (1.75)	135–149 (61–68)	141–158 (64–72)	150–175 (68–80)
5' 10" (1.78)	139–152 (63–69)	145–161 (66–73)	154–179 (70–81)
5' 11" (1.80)	143–155 (65–70)	149–165 (68–75)	159–183 (72–83)
6' (1.83)	147–159 (67–72)	153–169 (70–77)	163–187 (74–85)
6' 1" (1.85)	151–165 (69–75)	157–175 (71–80)	167–189 (76–86)
6' 2" (1.88)	155–168 (70–76)	161–179 (73–81)	171–197 (78–89)
6' 3" (1.90)	157–173 (72–79)	166–185 (75–84)	176–202 (80–92)

WOMEN

Height ft (m)	Small Frame lbs (kg)	Medium Frame lbs (kg)	Large Frame lbs (kg)
4' 10" (1.47)	91–108 (41–49)	95–115 (43–52)	103–119 (47–54)
4' 11" (1.50)	93–112 (42–51)	98–121 (44–55)	106–125 (48–57)
5' (1.52)	96–115 (44–52)	101–124 (46–57)	109–128 (49–58)
5' 1" (1.55)	99–118 (45–54)	104–127 (47–58)	112–131 (51–59)
5' 2" (1.57)	102–121 (46–55)	107–132 (49–60)	115–135 (52–61)
5' 3" (1.60)	105–124 (48–56)	110–135 (50–62)	118–138 (54–63)
5' 4" (1.63)	108–127 (49–58)	113–138 (51–63)	122–142 (55–65)
5' 5" (1.65)	111–130 (50–59)	117–141 (53–64)	126–145 (57–66)
5' 6" (1.68)	115–133 (52–60)	121–144 (55–66)	130–148 (59–67)
5' 7" (1.70)	119–136 (54–62)	125–147 (57–67)	134–151 (61–69)
5' 8" (1.73)	123–139 (56–63)	128–150 (58–68)	137–155 (62–71)
5' 9" (1.75)	127–142 (58–64)	133–153 (60–69)	141–159 (64–73)
5' 10" (1.78)	131–145 (59–66)	137–156 (62–71)	146–165 (66–75)
5' 11" (1.80)	135–148 (61–68)	141–159 (64–72)	150–170 (68–77)
6' (1.83)	138–151 (63–69)	143–163 (65–74)	153–173 (69–79)

paper. The upper arm should be flat on the paper with the forearm in the air at an angle of 90° at the elbow. Using the thumb and index finger of the other hand, find the bones on either side of the elbow at their widest point. Lower your fingers to the paper, making sure that you maintain the same distance between them and remove your arm. Then, with a pencil, mark the two points on the paper on the inside of your finger and thumb and measure the distance between them, preferably in centimetres. Although not entirely accurate, the measurement gives a reasonable indication of frame size.

Table 3 on page 62 gives the measurements of elbow width for women and men of medium frame at different heights. A larger measurement indicates a large frame and a smaller measurement, a small frame.

Having ascertained your frame size, table 4 on page 63, showing a reasonable weight range for people of different heights, can be used as a guide. The weights shown are those that are considered to be a standard range for young adults. As previously noted, middle-aged and older people tend to be heavier. Also, people who are athletes, those who carry out weight training or who play a lot of sport and so have developed a great deal of muscle, are heavier simply because muscle weighs more than fat! These factors emphasize the need to interpret the tables sensibly. You may be a little overweight according to the tables, but as long as your BMI lies within the healthy range, there is no medical reason for you to embark upon a diet.

Body shape

Finally, there is one other factor that can be taken in to account when deciding whether you need to lose weight and that is your body shape. There are two main types of body shape – apple and pear – and the category in which you belong is determined by your waist to hip ratio. Use a tape measure to obtain the figures, either in inches or centimetres, and divide the waist measurement by that of the hip. If the number obtained is less than 0.85 for women or 0.95 for men, then you are pear-shaped. If it is more, then you are apple-shaped. Apple-shaped people tend to store excess fat above the waist in their abdomen and this is the more usual pattern for men. Unfortunately, it is associated with a higher risk of the development of obesity-associated diseases and conditions such as heart and circulatory disease, high blood pressure, diabetes and elevated levels of blood cholesterol. The fact that more men than women have this body shape may be one of the reasons why men in western countries are susceptible to heart disease. However, once again, providing that your BMI lies within the healthy range there is no need to do more than endeavour to eat a good low fat diet and take regular exercise. Encouragingly, excess fat above the waist is fairly easy to lose and this is one of the reasons why men who diet are often quite successful.

Pear-shaped people store fat below the waist, around the hips and bottom and in the upper legs. In women, the fat stores here are utilised during pregnancy and breast-feeding and are part of the body's natural resources. For this reason, pear-shaped women often find it difficult to lose fat from these areas. When they go on a diet, they can discover (frustratingly!) that weight is lost above the waist, such as from the bust, where they may already be quite trim, before it starts to come off the desired areas of the hips and thighs. Pear-shaped people are also not immune to heart and circulatory disease and other conditions related to obesity. Hence, like the 'apples', it is sensible for 'pears' to eat a healthy, low-fat diet, incorporate as much exercise as possible into the daily routine and lose weight if BMI or other factors indicate that it is necessary to do so.

Blood cholesterol

Other factors which would indicate that a change of diet is necessary is a high level of blood cholesterol, as this is certainly a risk factor in the development of atheroma and atherosclerosis (furring of the arteries). As stated previously, a high level of blood cholesterol is related to the consumption of a western diet rich in saturated fats, with those who are overweight or obese known to be vulnerable (see Nutrition – Fats, page 14). However, the relationship with body weight is not necessarily a simple, straightforward one and it is possible for people who are not particularly overweight to have elevated blood cholesterol levels. The most accurate way to ascertain your level of cholesterol is by analysis of a blood sample, (although there are some 'over the counter' kits available from chemists and pharmacists). Most medical centres now run Well Woman and Well Man Clinics and a check on blood cholesterol levels is one of the preventative health care measures that is offered to patients. A regular health check-up is advisable for all middle-aged and older people but anyone can ask for their blood cholesterol level to be ascertained. Appropriate measures can then be taken, if the level is too high, to safeguard future health and this is very likely to include changes being made in the diet.

Hopefully, a consideration of all the factors discussed above can help you to decide whether you need to lose weight in order to safeguard your health, or whether you wish to do so in order to look and feel better about yourself. Additionally or alternatively, you may have decided that it is time to change to a healthier pattern of eating without necessarily expecting a reduction in weight. In fact several diet plans, especially those aiming for a long-term, slow loss of weight, fall more naturally into the latter category. These diet plans are concerned with showing people how to eat healthily so that their weight adjusts to its natural 'set point'. The set point is a person's optimum weight range, which varies around a median level by about ten pounds and is genetically determined. If you are already eating a sensible, healthy diet, are neither fat nor thin and find that your weight does not change very much, then it is likely to lie within the set point range. This factor helps to explain why it can be hard for a dieter to lose the final few pounds to achieve a pre-selected 'target' weight, which may simply have been placed too low for that person's individual set point weight range.

Basal metabolic rate (BMR)

As has been shown, actual weight depends upon a number of different factors, including food intake, lifestyle and amount of physical activity, genes, metabolism, age and existing medical conditions or health problems. The basal metabolic rate (BMR) is the amount of energy (calories) required by the body while at rest to perform the vital functions of heartbeat, respiration, maintenance of body temperature and cellular processes.

Rough calculation of BMR

It can be roughly calculated by multiplying your weight in pounds by a factor of 11, for adults in their twenties. For every decade beyond 20, 2 per cent of the total must be subtracted as this allows for the fact that metabolism slows down with ageing.

Example 1:
For example Suzanne weighs 9 stone 7 lbs and is aged 45:
133 lbs x 11 = 1463
2% of 1463 = 29.26
We now need to subtract 59 [i.e. 2 x 29.26] from 1463, 2% for every decade beyond the twenties.
Suzanne's BMR = 463–59 = <u>1404 kcals per day</u>

Example 2:
Brian weighs 12 stone 4 lbs and is aged 55.
168 lbs x 11 = 1848
2% of 1848 = 36.96
We now need to subtract 111 [i.e. 3 x 36.96] from 1848, 2% for every decade beyond the twenties.
Brian's BMR = <u>1737 kcals per day</u>

The Harris–Benedict Equation for BMR

Other factors can affect the BMR. The last calculation took age into account. Age brings less lean body mass and slows the BMR. Other factors include: the amount of the thyroid hormone thyroxin which is secreted (the more thyroxin the higher the BMR); growth (children and pregnant women have higher BMRs; body composition (the more lean tissue the higher the BMR) environmentatl temperature (heat and cold both raise the BMR).

Another method used to calculate BMR is known as the Harris–Benedict Equation. This takes height and sex into account. Sex is a differential because of the difference in body composition between men and women.

Males: 66 + (13.7 x W) + (5 x H) – (6.8 x A)
Females: 655 + (9.6 x W) + (1.7 x H) – (4.7 x A)
W stands for weight in kilograms (weight in pounds divided by 2.2).
H stands for height in centimetres (height in inches x 2.54).
A stands for age in years.

Suzanne weighs 9 stone 7 lbs (133lbs or 60 kg), she is 5 foot 6 inches tall (66 inches or 167.64 cm) and aged 45.
  W = 60, H = 167.64, A = 45
  655 + (9.6 x 60) + (1.7 x 167) – (4.7 x 45)
  655 + 576 + 284 – 211 = <u>1304 kcals per day</u>
Suzanne's friend Peter is the same height, weight and age as her but his BMR will be higher because he is a man and men have more lean muscle tissue and less body fat than women.
  66 + (13.7 x 60) + (5 x 167) – (6.8 x 45) = <u>1584 kcals per day</u>

Brian weighs 76 kg, is 5 foot 11 inches tall (180.34 cm), and is aged 55.
  66 + (13.7 x 76) + (5 x 180) – (6.8 x 55)
  66 + 1041.2 + 900 – 374 = <u>1633.2 kcals per day</u>

Brian's friend John is the same age and weight but is only 5 foot 3 inches tall. His BMR is 1533 <u>kcals per day</u>.

The above calculations are approximations. Of course, even the most sedentary person requires more calories than the amount demanded by BMR alone. All activity requires energy as fuel, including eating and digesting food – a process which temporarily raises the metabolic rate and burns up some calories to produce heat. Physical activity and regular exercise use up calories but the relationship is a more complex one than many people realize. While exercise plays a crucial part in successful dieting and, most importantly, producing a body that looks and feels good, unless one exercises very hard indeed, it is not a particularly good method of losing weight on its own. (See Exercise section on page 70).

It is known that there is a close relationship between BMR and weight and the heavier the body, the higher the BMR. It is estimated that BMR accounts for about two-thirds of the body's daily need for calories, with the remaining third required for all other activities, just to maintain the person at his or her current weight. Clearly, in order to lose weight, a person needs to eat fewer calories and, as has already been indicated, this may mean nothing more than making adjustments to the diet such as cutting out unnecessary and fattening snacks or second helpings! Many diet plans, especially those aimed at short-term weight loss, are based on a very limited intake of calories. Although this is probably all right for most people for a limited period, it is not a good idea to remain on such a stringent regime for very long. The best diets allow for a gradual return to normal, healthy eating once weight loss has been achieved which will maintain the person at his or her new weight.

Finally, all health experts agree that an average weight loss of 1 to 2 lbs each week should be the aim when dieting. Obviously, the amount of excess weight will determine the overall period of the diet, but it must also be borne in mind that the rate of loss is not uniform. Frequently, a greater amount of weight is lost at the start of a diet (but see Physical Aspects of Weight Loss on page 69) than towards the end, so it is necessary to be both patient and persistent. It is always worth remembering that a slow, steady loss of weight is much more likely to result in long-term success, particularly if you remain determined!

Physical Aspects of Weight Loss – How the Body Reacts to Dieting

AN understanding of the way the body reacts when food intake is restricted is helpful for anyone who is thinking of going on a diet. The body stores energy in the form of glycogen (animal starch) which is a complex, polysaccharide carbohydrate that is found in liver and muscle cells. If food intake is insufficient to supply the necessary amount of glucose for energy needs, the body turns first to its glycogen stores. Each glycogen molecule incorporates a considerable quantity of water into its structure. This is released by hydrolysis in order to make the glucose part of the molecule available to the body for its shortfall in energy. Water is heavy and during the first week of a diet, three to four pints of it (up to 2.3 litres) are eliminated from the body, as glycogen stores are utilised. This amount of water weighs 3 to 4 lbs (up to 1.8 kg) and accounts for most of the initial 'weight' loss of a diet, but no fat has as yet been eliminated! If you stop the diet after one week, the water (and the weight) is immediately reclaimed as the body replenishes its glycogen stores. It is only as the diet continues that the body begins to utilise its fat stores and this is a much slower process which, as has already been stated, is best achieved at a rate of 1 to 2 lbs (450 to 900 g) per week.

It is important to realize that the body's reaction to a restricted intake of food is to lower the metabolic rate so that fewer calories are required for daily energy needs. This process happens quite quickly and is a physiological survival mechanism, evolved to ensure that life will be prolonged for as long as possible during times of food shortage. Hence, the body reacts to a restricted calorie intake by attempting to conserve its reserves of fat and other tissue. This explains why it can be quite a difficult and slow process to utilise and use up your stores of fat, especially if you are not particularly overweight. Another factor which must be taken into account is that the body utilises muscle and other lean tissue, as well as fat, to provide energy during a diet. This is much more likely to happen if dieting is extreme and so emphasis should be on the importance of adopting a sensible and sustainable approach to losing weight. At the rate of a pound or so a week, loss of lean tissue is minimal and in accordance with the amount of fat being lost. Exercising during dieting helps to preserve muscle and burn up calories and the more lean tissue there is compared to fat, the higher the metabolic rate. Hence exercise can help to counter the natural fall in metabolic rate which accompanies dieting. In general, it will take about three months or so to lose a stone in weight but this varies between different people, according to individual characteristics and the nature of the diet. Once the target weight has been reached and a normal pattern of eating is resumed, the metabolic rate adjusts to its new level. It is normal for a little weight to be regained at the end of the period of dieting but this is water rather than fat and is connected with the body's replenishment of its glycogen stores.

Exercise

There is universal agreement among health experts about the benefits of regular exercise in promoting and maintaining good health and in aiding weight loss during dieting. Exercise helps to relieve various common disorders such as hypertension, depression and constipation and helps to prevent the heart and circulatory diseases that are so prevalent among people in western countries. For all people, even those suffering from certain chronic conditions, exercising within the limits of their strength makes them feel better and promotes restful sleep. The forms and benefits of exercise are discussed in more detail on pages 75 to 76.

Regular physical exercise is vital throughout life to help maintain good health and to confer the ability to remain active, even in old age. Exercise burns up some of the calories in food and so reduces the availability of any excess being laid down as fat. During dieting, exercise uses up a greater proportion of the calories that are consumed so that the body has to turn to its fat stores to provide energy. Fat is naturally deposited and stored in muscle, particularly if muscles are not being properly used. Exercise prevents and reverses this process, increasing the bulk of muscle and using the fat stores as fuel. Muscles are metabolically active even while at rest, so by ensuring that the body has plenty of muscle through regular exercise, more calories are utilised. Exercise confers a sense of well-being, promotes healthy sleep and makes the heart and circulation, lungs and respiration work more efficiently. It also gives you a good appetite, which can be a disadvantage for someone who is dieting and trying to restrict the amount of food being eaten! Vigorous exercise trains the heart so that the muscle fibres become stronger and pump a greater volume of blood with each beat. The result of this is that the resting heartbeat rate slows down and the system works more efficiently. This is achieved by regular, fairly hard activity (called aerobic exercise) which is sufficient to raise the heart and respiration rate for about 15 to 20 minutes, carried out three times each week (or more frequently or for longer, once a person becomes fit). Through its beneficial effects upon the heart and circulation, this type of exercise helps to lower blood pressure, hence reducing the incidence of problems arising from this condition.

Regular exercise training of this sort raises the basal metabolic rate (BMR) which means that the number of calories used while the body is at rest (for respiration, heartbeat, digestion, organ tissue and cell function) is increased. This is one of the great benefits for a dieter since it means that calories from food are more likely to be used and so weight loss is promoted. Non-aerobic 'strength' exercises, particularly some forms of weight-bearing activities, pump calcium into bones and help maintain their density and strength. In older age, this has been shown to significantly reduce the rate at which bone density is lost, hence lessening the risk of fractures.

In summary, different types of exercise and activity can improve bodily health in three main ways:

1 Stamina, fitness or endurance is the ability to sustain a period of vigorous activity without having to stop because your heart is racing and you are gasping for breath! This is built up gradually by an aerobic exercise regime that trains the heart, circulation, lungs and respiration in the manner outlined above. An improvement in fitness is usually noticed quite quickly, after three or four weeks of regular, fairly hard activity and this provides a great encouragement to continue! Unfortunately, however, the level of fitness soon declines if the exercise regime is abandoned, so having worked to make the gains, it is worthwhile to make the effort and find the time to continue. Aerobic exercise, such as vigorous walking, jogging, cycling, dancing, hill walking and many sports – football, tennis, netball, basketball, squash, badminton, etc. – all help to get you fit.

2 Flexibility is the ability of the muscles to perform their full range of movements – twisting, flexing and stretching – with suppleness and

ease. There are many exercises that are designed to improve the flexibility and tone of various muscles and joints in different parts of the body and numerous books and videos are available. For example, many yoga exercises come in to this category. Health practitioners and sports club instructors are normally happy to advise upon the type of exercises that would be of greatest benefit to each individual. Such exercises, which involve stretching, bending and 'loosening up' should always be performed before and after vigorous aerobic activities and sports in order to lessen the risk of injuries or cramps.

3 Strength exercises are aimed at increasing the tone and sometimes the bulk of muscles, leading to the firming up of the body and an improvement in appearance and posture. This reshaping process can, if required, be targeted onto individual trouble spots such as the upper arms, thighs, bottom and stomach. Callanetics, weight training and specially designed gym equipment come into this category but so do a whole series of simple exercises which can be performed at home. Once again, there are many books available on these types of exercises and health and fitness instructors are usually happy to give individual advice. However, anyone who is very unfit or overweight, has an existing medical condition or is aged over 35 is advised to obtain a doctor's advice before attempting to use weights or gym equipment.

Most people recognize the need to undertake physical exercise but for many a perceived lack of free time makes it difficult for them to fit this into their daily routine. People also commonly make the mistake of launching into a fast, vigorous or 'extreme' form of exercise when they are not at all fit to do so. This can be dangerous if there is any underlying, undiagnosed condition such as heart disease or a back or joint problem and may cause illness or injury. In any exercise regime, it is important to be sensible and to increase the level of activity as and when fitness improves. Most vital of all is to stop if it hurts! Contrary to popular belief, pain in exercise is not good for you but is the body's way of telling you that you are doing too much.

People who are prepared to take a critical look at their daily routine usually find that there are slots in their schedule where some physical activity can be fitted in, without causing undue disruption. A well-known and often-quoted example of this is to use the stairs, rather than the lift, at work and to park the car further away in order to fit in a brisk walk or run. It is important to realize that even small measures such as these have a beneficial effect and help to improve fitness, using up some calories and providing a base from which to progress to other forms of exercise. Several routine home activities equally fall into this category including cleaning and vacuuming, decorating and DIY, gardening and mowing the lawn because various muscles are being made to work and the person is actively moving about.

As mentioned on page 72, it is advisable for anyone aged over 35 years or who is overweight to check with a doctor before embarking upon a vigorous form of exercise. You should stop if the activity causes discomfort or pain or if you are fighting for breath. Do not exercise hard soon after eating a meal. It is best to eat a starchy meal, which will provide plenty of energy, about three hours before exercising and to drink plenty of water before, during and after the period of activity. You should avoid exercise if you have any form of illness, particularly if you are feverish or anaemic. If you suffer from any form of chronic illness or condition, exercise in accordance with medical advice. Always make sure that you are wearing the correct clothing, footwear and headgear appropriate for the activity and that it is of good quality and fits well. Injuries are often caused through neglect in this area and the cost of equipment is a factor that needs to be taken into account when choosing an exercise or activity.

Finally and most importantly, choose an activity that you enjoy and that is appropriate for you, even if it lies outside the usual range of fitness and exercise regimes. For example, if you enjoy gardening, make this a priority and if your own garden does not present a sufficient challenge how about offering to cut an elderly neighbour's grass? Voluntary and local organisations are always looking for willing, active people to help with a whole range of activities – from maintaining paths to minor (or major!) DIY projects or with helping to set up, and clear up after a fête, fair or show. All this involves active exercise, even if it is different to that being offered by the local health and fitness centre, and usually has the added benefit of being enjoyable from a social pint of view. Certainly, the social aspect of exercise is something else to take into consideration when making a choice of activity – at a dance or karate class or when playing a team sport, you are likely to make new friends.

Although this may seem obvious, people can be influenced by many factors, including what others may say or do and hence do not always make wise choices. Of course, there is no harm in trying a sport or type of exercise to see if you like it, but be prepared to give it up if you do not.

The important factor in this case is not to be discouraged but to try something else, rather than thinking that exercise is just not right for you! You are far more likely to succeed in the activity and hence to improve your level of fitness if you enjoy it and look forward to the times when you can carry it out. Dieters have the added bonus of knowing that they are helping themselves to lose weight. Ex-dieters can feel secure in the knowledge that exercising helps the lost pounds to remain that way! But best of all, everyone, whatever their age, weight or shape can be sure that by exercising, they are taking a positive step towards safeguarding their health both for the present and into the future.

The chart on pages 75 and 76 can be used to give you an idea of how many calories (in relation to body weight) you are likely to use when engaged in a variety of activities and exercise.

Overdoing it – a word of warning

Usually, exercise of any sort generates a feeling of wellbeing which is one of the reasons why it is so valuable in the treatment of depression. Hard physical exercise can cause an even more intense experience of elation and exhilaration – an 'exercise high' – which is believed to result from the release of protein substances called endorphins from the pituitary gland at the base of the brain. These are involved in hormonal activity and also have pain-relieving qualities similar to those of morphine. They are released during times of physical stress, as in hard exercise, and it is believed that in these circumstances they cause the feelings of pleasurable exhilaration. Some health experts are concerned that those who regularly exercise hard may be in danger of causing damage to their body in order to achieve this feeling of elation. They may be ignoring warning signs such as pain and may, in some respects, be addicted to the 'exercise high'. Exercising can then become compulsive – something that the person feels that he or she must do, often at the expense of other aspects of life. Compulsive exercising is also a risk factor in eating disorders. If you, or someone you know, comes into this category then it is time to examine what is happening, possibly by talking to a health professional. There is growing evidence that regularly punishing the body with stressful, hard physical exercise is as damaging as not exercising at all. Sudden, unexpected deaths have been reported among those who come into this category and there is increasing concern that these people may suffer damage to organs, skeletal muscle and tendons, which damage which may cause them serious problems in middle and older age.

Table 5: Number of calories burned in 30 minutes of activity (in relation to body weight)

Activity/ exercise	50 kg	55 kg	60kg	65 kg	70 kg	75 kg
Aerobics	155	170	186	200	225	250
Badminton	190	200	210	220	230	240
Basketball	310	350	390	430	470	500
Bowling	95	100	105	110	115	120
Canoeing	120	125	135	140	145	150
Carpentry	125	135	140	145	150	160
Cooking	70	75	80	85	90	95
Cycling	150	165	180	195	210	240
Dancing, moderate	115	120	130	135	140	150
Dancing, fast	300	310	320	330	340	350
Dish-washing	70	75	80	085	90	95
Dressing	40	40	45	45	50	50
Driving	50	55	60	65	70	75
Exercise, moderate	150	160	170	180	190	200
Exercise, fast	200	220	240	260	280	300
Football	275	300	325	350	375	400
Gardening	120	130	140	150	160	170
Golf, no cart	120	125	130	140	145	150
Golf, with cart	70	75	80	85	90	95
Handball	260	275	290	310	330	350
Hockey (field or ice)	300	310	320	330	340	350
Horse-back riding	130	140	150	160	170	180
Housework, active	100	105	110	120	125	135
Ironing	70	70	75	75	80	80
Jogging, light	225	235	245	255	265	275
Lacrosse	300	315	330	345	360	375
Office work	65	70	75	80	85	90

Activity/ exercise	50 kg	55 kg	60kg	65 kg	70 kg	5 kg
Painting (walls)	130	135	140	150	160	170
Piano playing	100	105	110	115	120	125
Reading	15	15	20	20	25	25
Rowing	325	350	375	400	425	450
Running, slow	290	315	345	375	405	435
Running, fast	375	415	450	490	525	550
Sewing	25	25	30	30	35	35
Singing	35	40	45	50	55	60
Sitting at rest	15	15	20	20	25	25
Skating, energetically	250	260	270	280	290	300
Skiing, energetically	250	260	270	280	290	300
Stair climbing	170	185	200	215	230	250
Sweeping floor	70	75	80	90	100	110
Swimming, slow	190	210	230	250	270	290
Swimming, fast	240	260	285	305	330	355
Tennis	165	180	195	215	230	245
Typing	85	90	95	100	105	110
Volleyball	170	185	200	215	230	250
Walking, moderately	105	115	125	135	145	155
Walking, fast	125	135	145	155	165	175
Writing	50	55	60	65	70	75

Starting a Diet –
Points to Consider

IF you have decided that you wish to begin dieting, there are a few points which it is helpful to consider first and which should aid your eventual success. The first question is whether it is appropriate for you to go it alone or whether you should seek the advice of your doctor before you embark upon a diet. As previously stated, a doctor's advice is essential if you have a BMI of 30 or above or suffer from an existing medical condition. Your doctor may wish to refer you to a dietician who will help to devise a diet plan appropriate for you and will provide follow-up appointments to monitor your progress.

You should not diet at all if your BMI is less than 20. If you are aged under 18 and feel that you need to lose weight, it is essential for you to consult your doctor so that you will receive appropriate advice. At this age you are still growing and any diet that you embark upon must contain all the nutritional elements that are necessary for normal growth and development. Pregnant women should not diet and neither should nursing mothers – you will certainly receive advice from health professionals about healthy eating during this time! Finally, if you have tried to diet in the past but have been unsuccessful, or feel so unhappy about your weight that it is interfering with everyday life, consulting your doctor will almost certainly provide reassurance. If you can, make an appointment at a Well Woman or Well Man clinic so that you can ask advice about your weight, along with any other health concerns that you may have.

The next stage involves some honest self-examination to identify your individual motives and goals in dieting. If you are prepared to look thoroughly at yourself, as you are now, you will obtain an honest personal appraisal which will help you to choose the type of diet plan that is right for you. The sort of questions that you should ask yourself are listed below and you may be able to add others of your own!

1 What are your motives for dieting and what do you expect life to be like for the new, slimmer you compared with that of the person you are today? If your answer is that slimming will make you feel fitter and generally more positive about yourself then that is fine.

  If, on the other hand, you expect great changes such as becoming more attractive to the opposite sex, being happier and generally finding more opportunities opening up to you then beware. These things have undoubtedly happened for some people who have shed weight, especially for those who were originally obese. However, others have found that life has continued in much the same way as before or that they have even had to contend with new problems such as jealousy in a partner or close friend.

2 Are you dieting for yourself or in order to please or fulfil the expectations of others? (The 'others' in this context may simply be the media or fashion industries who relentlessly promote the idea of thinness, exerting subtle pressure on countless normal-sized people who are made to feel inadequate).

  Research shows that those who are dieting for themselves but with the encouragement of family and friends, are far more likely to be motivated to succeed. Sometimes a person is put under pressure to diet by a partner or family members when he or she does not see the need to do so. If someone is very overweight or obese, then those close to that person may well feel worried or concerned upon health grounds.

  However, sometimes the pressure, particularly from a partner, amounts to nothing more than emotional blackmail and is far-removed from loving concern. Anyone whose partner threatens to withhold social treats, holidays, new clothes, etc, or who makes the person feel unworthy of love and affection because of his or her weight, is engaging in this nasty and unhelpful practice, which is selfishly motivated and cruel. If you find yourself on the receiving end of this kind of treatment, examine your relationship along with whether you wish to diet. Dieting should always be a matter of individual, personal choice, even for those who are obese since, in the final analysis, each person has to take responsibility for his or her own health. The role of health professionals is to provide information and that of family and friends to encourage and never to coerce.

3 What are your current eating habits, likes and dislikes? You may be the sort of person who finds it easy to stick to three meals a day, with nothing in between, or who prefers to eat a little and often. You may find it difficult to resist high calorie snacks such as crisps, chocolate, sweets and biscuits or you may eat a good breakfast, skip lunch and last until dinner in the evening. Are you able to eat less during the week but like to be more indulgent when relaxing at the weekend? Do you feel that you would wish to include the occasional alcoholic drink in your diet? Are you the sort of person who cannot bear to waste food and so you finish up left-overs rather than throwing them out?

4 Are you just preparing meals for yourself or for a partner and family? If you are cooking for several people, you will need to consider whether you can be bothered to prepare separate dishes for yourself, as may be required by some diet plans. If this is going to be difficult, then you may wish to just select items from the family menu that are suitable for a weight-loss diet.

5   Are you happy to count and add up calories and to weigh portions of food? Many diets require you to do one or both of these things and this can take some getting used to, especially at the beginning.

6 Are you wanting a short or a long-term diet and how much weight do you wish to lose? As has already been mentioned, the most successful diets are those that allow for a slow, steady weight loss over a fairly prolonged period. However, sometimes a person just wishes to lose a small amount of weight for a particular occasion – and there are diet plans that are quite suitable for this.

7   Would you prefer a very exact, rigid type of diet or one which is a little more flexible? Some diet plans set out the foods to be eaten each day in minute detail, which can be quite irritating or helpful, depending upon individual point of view. Some diets allow for a between-meal snack, even if this is only a raw carrot or a stick of celery and this may be more suitable for those who feel that they would like to have something to stave off any pangs of hunger!

8 Does the idea of slimming with other people appeal to you or fill you with horror? As with so many other aspects of life, the support and encouragement of other like-minded people can be a great help to those who are dieting and meeting with others turns slimming into a social activity, at least to a certain extent. There is no doubt that the large slimming organisations, such as Weight Watchers, are highly successful and help many people to lose weight, providing not only the diet plans but friendly and professional help and advice. They provide a useful service but one which is by no means inexpensive and hence a further question to be taken into consideration is:

9 What is the cost of the diet? It is not only slimming clubs that can work out to be costly. Several other diets, including those in which one buys specific products as in meal replacement plans, or those which demand exotic or expensive items, can work out to be expensive too. Hence it is well worth considering the overall cost of a diet plan but do not despair if you are on a limited budget – dieting should only reduce the pounds on your waistline and not the ones in your wallet or purse!

Answering these sorts of questions honestly will help you examine the range of diets in the next section of this book with a critical eye, in order to pick out one which is best suited to your aspirations and lifestyle.

Tips for successful dieting and for staying slim

There are several ways in which you can help yourself to successfully lose weight and prevent it from coming back once you have finished dieting. As has been seen, the reasons for being overweight can be varied and complex but, for many people in the West, it is simply a matter of consuming too many calories in the form of fat and taking too little exercise. Hence, first and foremost, recognize that your present diet and lifestyle are unsatisfactory, as far as your weight is concerned, and must be changed if you wish to meet with success. Aim to reduce, forever, the amount of fat that you consume and do not gradually slip back into former ways of eating once you have finished dieting. This does not mean that you can never eat high-fat foods, but just that you must have them occasionally rather than frequently.

Drink plenty of water. A glass of water before a meal will help to fill the stomach and reduce the amount of food eaten. The same effect can be gained by eating some salad vegetables (celery, lettuce, cucumber, raw carrot, tomato, etc) before eating a meal. Always keep plenty of salad vegetables and fruit available so that if you do feel hungry, you have a low-calorie, healthy snack on hand. Eat plenty of green vegetables – they are good for you and contain very few calories. Chew your food thoroughly and eat slowly, however hungry you are. Research has shown that it takes 20 minutes for the brain to register a feeling of fullness from the stomach so, if you eat quickly, you will consume more than you need before you feel full. Stop eating at the point when you feel that you could manage just a little more and aim to be satisfied but not over-full. Try to take more exercise, even if only in simple ways, both during and after dieting. As has been seen, exercise is vital both for good health and for weight control and for shaping and toning the body.

One of the difficulties faced by a dieter is what to do when asked out to a dinner party where, more often than not, high calorie food is likely to be served. There are several strategies that can be employed to enable dieters to enjoy social occasions without taking their weight control programme too badly off course. If you know your host/hostess well, a phone call in advance of the event should enable you to ask if you can select items from the menu that are suitable for your diet, without causing offence. This is usually easier and less embarrassing than trying to refuse food that has already been prepared once you are seated at the dinner table. If you do not know your hosts well, then it is obviously more difficult and you may not feel up to explaining that you are on a diet.

Possibly the best approach is to ask for small portions of all that is offered, as it is easier to plead a small appetite than a diet. If you feel that your self-control may falter if faced with an array of high calorie food, then do not worry too much. Even if you do eat more than you intended, you can compensate for this by following a slightly stricter regime for a few days before and/or after the dinner party. Eating out in a restaurant is somewhat easier for a dieter because it is generally possible to select a meal compatible with a weight loss programme.

For those who have reached their desired weight and are no longer dieting, following the strategies outlined above should help to ensure that they remain slim. However, many people find it helpful to follow 'the 5 lbs rule'. This involves continuing to weigh yourself once each week as you did when you were dieting. If your weight creeps up to 5 lbs (2.27 kg) beyond your target weight, resume your diet until the excess has been lost. In this way, you should be able to control your weight without having to embark upon a long-term diet once again. Feel encouraged by the fact that very many people are successful in maintaining their weight loss, or only regain a little once they cease to diet rather than returning to their former size – and there is no reason why you should not be one of them!

11

Diets Guide

In this section of the book, a number of popular and effective diets are described which cover a wide variety of lifestyles and food preferences. Whether you are a vegetarian, find it hard to cook, do or do not wish to count calories, there should be a diet here to suit you. For example, if your sweet tooth is your downfall we have the Chocoholics Diet, if you need a low fat regime incorporated with an exercise programme then there is Rosemary Conley's Hip and Thigh Diet, or for those who need to curb a voracious appetite there is the G-Index Diet.

Each section describes how the diets work, who they are best suited to and the speed at which weight loss can be achieved. A sample daily menu for each diet is provided, where appropriate, and there are also publishers' details to enable you to find the books and follow the entire diets if you so wish.

Faddy diets are no substitute for sustained healthy eating and exercise. The diets listed here contain advice which may be of inspiration in helping you to find a regime that suits you, however, always keep in mind the basic advice on good nutrition outlined in part one of this book.

The Body-clock Diet

USING research into female biorhythms, the Body-clock Diet is a weight loss programme which is designed to fit in with the chemical fluctuations that occur in women's bodies throughout the menstrual cycle.

Recommended for
It is recommended for women who experience symptoms such as mood swings, food cravings, increases in appetite and fluid retention – all of which are associated with premenstrual syndrome (PMS). These symptoms are usually experienced during the seven days leading up to the beginning of menstruation. However, research has shown that many women experience physical and psychological changes up to fourteen days before their period is due to start. Naturally, trying to sustain a diet when you are feeling depressed and moody or when you feel an irresistible urge for a chocolate bar can be extremely difficult.

Not recommended for
It is not recommended for men; women who are going through or have already been through the menopause; women who are pregnant or breastfeeding or who are trying to conceive.

Over a 24-hour period there are chemical fluctuations in the body that will affect mood, energy levels, appetite, the metabolism and blood-sugar levels. These fluctuations, known as 'biorhythms', can be profoundly affected by the hormones oestrogen and progesterone which govern the menstrual cycle, resulting in the symptoms of PMS. The degree to which these are experienced is dependent upon the individual's cycle; thus some women can experience an overwhelming urge for sugary foods several times a day, for up to two weeks before they are due to start their period. For other women the urge for something sweet may not be so strong and may be experienced only for the few days prior to menstruation.

Irrespective of the individual differences, many women on a diet would agree that typical slimming foods – fruit, vegetables and low-fat foods – will neither satisfy these cravings nor their increased hunger. So the premenstrual phase is often a time when diets are broken and the dieter feels that she is back to square one.

Carbohydrates in the form of simple sugars (e.g., chocolate, sweets) or in their more complex form (bread, potatoes, pasta, biscuits) are broken down rapidly during the digestive process (though this is more delayed in the case of complex carbohydrates). They give an immediate boost to the blood-glucose levels, satisfying both the hunger and the craving. However, this boost is not sustained and the cravings tend to be satisfied for a short period only.

The Body-clock Diet provides a questionnaire which enables the dieter to identify the nature of her own cycle and choose the diet plan which will be most appropriate for her. There are three diet plans based on a daily calorific intake from which the slimmer can choose:

• Plan 1000 – providing 1000 calories a day, it is recommended for women with 14 lb (6.3 kg) or less to lose.
• Plan 1250 – providing 1250 calories a day, it is recommended for women with 14 to 42 lb (6.3 to 19 kg) to lose.
• Plan 1500 – providing 1500 calories a day, it is recommended for women with 42 lb (19 kg) or more to lose.

Each diet plan is divided into three phases, each of which has a different calorie content and nutritional balance to match the changing body chemistry throughout the complete menstrual cycle. The first phase provides a dietary plan for the first part of the menstrual cycle from the first day of menstruation to around day fourteen. The calorie content is lowest during this phase and the emphasis placed on fruits and vegetables and starchy foods which have a high fibre content. In the second phase the menus feature predominantly low-fat foods with small amounts of sugary, starchy foods also included. In the third phase, the seven days immediately prior to a period when the mood swings, food cravings and increased appetite tend to be more prevalent, the daily calorific allowance is increased to enable the dieter to eat more sugary and starchy foods.

Each plan features a breakfast, a light meal and a main meal option with an added 100 calorie fruit allowance in the first phase. In the second phase an extra 100 calories allowance is made, to be chosen from fruit or from a list of suggested sugary and starchy treats for the Plan 1000 and the Plan 1250, while on the Plan 1500 the allowance for these treats is

250 calories. In the third phase the calorific allowance for extra snacks is set at between 300 and 750 calories, depending on which plan the dieter has chosen as the most appropriate.

A typical day's menu

A typical day's diet from Phase A on the Plan 1000 would be as follows:

Breakfast

1 boiled egg

1 rye crispbread smeared with low-fat spread

Light meal

1 wholemeal pitta bread with 50 g (2 oz) hummus and 6 stoned black olives (in brine) served with a salad from the allowance for unlimited vegetables

Main meal

Mushroom omelette served with salad and oil-free dressing and a piece of fruit from the allowance or sausage hotpot and a piece of fruit from the allowance

The flexibility of this programme enables the dieter to tailor the phases to her own needs. Thus, if you tend to experience food cravings only in the last seven days of your cycle you can stick to the first (and lowest) calorific phase of the diet for a longer period. The only rules are that you start the diet at the first phase on the first day of your period or as near to that day as possible. As menstruation begins the hormonal balance is restored to a state whereby the typical PMS cravings and hunger have diminished, making it the best time to maximise on a reduced food consumption. While in one phase you should not choose any of the menu options from the other phases as this will upset the nutritional balance that has been carefully devised for each phase.

Over 50 calorie-counted recipes are provided both for keen cooks and for the dieter who is short of time and needs easy-to-prepare options. There is also a good choice of recipes and meal suggestions for vegetarian slimmers.

Eating out

There is no specific advice for eating out.

How fast is it?

The author cites that an average weight loss on the Plan 1250 over a

28-day period is 9.8 lb (4.4 kg); this figure is based on the experience of dieters who kept the Body-clock plan for at least eight weeks and includes fluid loss as well as fat loss.

Exercise

The Body-clock diet also features an exercise programme, again divided into three phases to correspond to the stages of the menstrual cycle. This takes account of the fact that during the final phase of the cycle many women may experience a general lack of energy and disinclination to take part in physical activity. Each of the three exercise programmes feature exercises based on stretching, toning and aerobic movement to increase stamina, suppleness and strength. In addition, a chart of exercises from aerobics to yoga is provided giving the relative effects of each for stamina, suppleness and strength and the calorific expenditure per ten minutes.

Extras

The diet has a carefully devised readjustment programme which, once the dieter has reached her target weight, will enable her to increase her calorific intake gradually, without the classic pitfall of post-diet weight gain.

The positive philosophy behind the Body-clock Diet is that it is balanced with your body's individual monthly cycle and your lifestyle.

Full information about this diet is published in *The Body-clock Diet* by Dr Alan Maryon Davies (Network Books, 1996) £4.99.

The Chocoholic Diet

THE Chocoholic Diet is a low-fat, reduced-calorie weight loss programme that includes an allowance for chocolate treats. Furthermore, the diet plan encourages the chocolate addict to consider his or her attitude to chocolate – such as whether it is used at times of stress or emotional upset – and provides practical advice which can help turn a chocoholic into a healthy eater who enjoys the occasional chocolate snack.

Recommended for
It is recommended for anyone who wishes to lose weight but has always found that their chocolate addiction prevents significant success in dieting.

While alcohol and drugs are recognised as addictive, a persistent craving for chocolate might be laughed off as pure self-indulgence. However, chocolate does contain substances which can be regarded as addictive. Firstly, when chocolate is consumed the high content of refined sugar creates an immediate rush of energy as the body's blood-glucose level is suddenly boosted. This in turn initiates a release of insulin to control the blood-glucose balance, which will result in hunger or the desire to snack again. Caffeine and the substances theobromine and tyrosine, all of which are commonly found in chocolate, can exacerbate this imbalance, often leading to the craving sensation that only a chocolaty treat can satisfy.

The stimulant effects are not just restricted to blood-glucose levels. The chemical phenylethylanine, again a common ingredient in chocolate, is actually produced by the brain when we are in love – this has led to theories that chocolate can be used as a substitute for sex or emotional affection.

By consumption per head of population, the UK is the third highest consumer of chocolate in the world – which means a large number of people indulge their passion for chocolate more than is, perhaps, healthy for them. Quite apart from the high sugar content, chocolate is high in fat and a persistent consumption will, in all likelihood, lead to excessive weight gain over a period of time.

It is not surprising that many chocoholics will find dieting quite impossible; not only do they have to cope with a lower intake of food but they also have to contend with very real cravings which are both physical and psychological.

The Chocoholic Diet works on two levels, addressing the need to lose pounds and encouraging the dieter to analyse his or her relationship with chocolate on a more emotional and psychological level. To begin the diet the individual is asked to respond to a questionnaire that will identify what type of chocoholic they are. There are six categories:

- The Romantic – somebody who uses food for comfort and often indulges in chocolate as a substitute for love, affection and sex.
- The Secret Binger – somebody who indulges their passion for chocolate in secret, often refusing chocolate in public but consuming large amounts in private.
- The Comfort Eater – perhaps the most common type of chocoholic, comfort eaters often resort to chocolate when confronted with various pressures in their lives.
- The Weekend Indulger – those who use the weekends and holidays to indulge their passion for chocolaty foods.
- The Sugar Addict – those who eat chocolate in response to real physical stimuli.
- The Premenstrual Craver – women who experience cravings for highly-refined sugary foods as a symptom of PMS.

There is a diet plan for each of these six types of chocoholic, individually devised to meet dietary needs and to encourage dieters to find ways of coping with the feelings which have driven them to reach for the chocolate bar.

The diets are based around wholesome, filling carbohydrate foods such as baked potatoes, fruits, vegetables and salads in combination with lean protein foods, such as low-fat dairy products, skinless chicken and lean red meats.

For the first week of each plan chocolate is forbidden; in subsequent weeks, however, a calorie allowance is made for a chocolate confectionery or a chocolate snack to be chosen from recipes for small cakes, biscuits, desserts and drinks. The plan for Week 1 for the Secret Binger would be based on one breakfast, two light meals, one main meal and one treat. In the second week the plan would be the same with the addition of a 150 calorie allowance for chocolate and a 200 calorie allowance for one of the recipes.

The diet can then be continued in this way until the desired weight has been reached.

How fast is it?
By following the Chocoholic Diet plan the dieter should achieve a healthy, gradual weight loss.

Extras
An important part of the Chocoholic Diet is involved in encouraging the dieter to enjoy chocolate as a treat, as opposed to relying on it as a form of comfort or resorting to it in moments of stress. Practical advice is given for developing new techniques for coping with everyday situations, such as the pressure of deadlines at work or feelings of loneliness and isolation.

Full information about this diet is published in *The Chocoholic Diet Book* by Sally Ann Voak (Blake Paperbacks, 1992) £3.99.

Rosemary Conley's Complete Flat Stomach Plan

THE Complete Flat Stomach Plan is a four-week weight loss programme that specifically targets the problem of excess fat on the abdominal area and the waist through a low-fat diet and an exercise plan.

Recommended for

Those who wish to lose weight in the abdominal region. Those who need a diet with a 'little and often' approach.

Not recommended for

It is not recommended for anybody who feels the need to lose weight generally as opposed to spot reducing. General weight loss will be achieved on this diet but the exercise programme is devised especially for toning stomach muscles.

Based on low-fat foods, the eating plan has been devised around guidelines and menus that will provide the dieter with three meals a day. The diet can also be used by people who do not enjoy cooking or do not have much time for food preparation, as a list of recommended low-fat ready meals is included. The one basic rule of the programme is that the dieter eats all three meals but, as far as possible, avoids snacking during the day. There is a list of forbidden foods which includes all confectionery, cakes and biscuits, oils and fats (excepting those that have been fat reduced to four per cent or less), cheese (except low-fat cottage cheese), fried foods and fatty meats and meat products such as sausages and pâté.

Before starting the eating plan, the dieter is given practical advice on how to set realistic goals and how to cope with 'bad diet days' and resume weight-loss objectives.

The eating plan is well-balanced, varied and imaginative, consisting of breakfast, lunch and an evening meal which includes a starter, a main course and a dessert. The breakfast option can be chosen from three categories: Cereals, Fruit-based Breakfasts or Cooked and Continental breakfasts. The lunches include choices from salads, sandwiches, jacket potatoes, branded foods and gourmet options – the flexibility here caters for those who need packed lunches. The evening meal options are also tailored to individual needs with quick and easy recipes, recommended convenience meals, vegetarian choices and gourmet recipes.

A typical day's menu
Daily allowance
450 ml (^{3}/$_4$ pint) skimmed or semi-skimmed milk

150 ml (^{1}/$_4$ pint) unsweetened fruit juice

One unit of alcohol for women; two units for men

Unlimited tea and coffee (using milk from the daily allowance), water and low-calorie carbonated drinks

Unlimited salad and vegetables, cooked without fat

Breakfast
50 g (2 oz) cornflakes with 1 teaspoon of sugar and 115 g (4 oz) of fresh fruit

Lunch
Sandwich made with 2 large slices of wholemeal bread with a filling of 1 hard-boiled egg mixed with 1 tablespoon of low-fat yoghurt or fat-reduced salad dressing

or

Marks & Spencer pasta salad with sweetcorn, plus 1x150 g (5 oz) diet yoghurt

Dinner
Crudités served with a garlic and mint yoghurt dip as a starter

Beef and mushroom kebabs *or* spinach and pasta bake *or* chicken pilaf as a main course

1 pot Cadbury's light low-fat chocolate mousse

or

Strawberry layer dessert

Eating out
Basic practical advice is given for enjoying a meal out while on the programme. This includes tips for reading the menu carefully, asking staff

for advice about ingredients, requesting that vegetables be prepared without fat and beginning the meal with a long low-calorie drink, to assuage the appetite a little.

How fast is it?

There are no specific averages or expectations for weight or inch loss. However, the statistics from the original 1000-strong diet team that tested the programme are very encouraging. In responding to questionnaires a remarkable 98.4 per cent reported that they had lost weight and inches; 71.3 per cent lost most of the inches from the waist and the abdomen and 95 per cent said that they enjoyed the diet. The average weight loss for those who had stuck strictly to the diet was just over 10 lb (4.5 kg) over a four week period.

Exercise

The exercise programme has been devised for three levels of ability and activity – Elementary, Intermediate and Advanced. These toning exercises are designed specifically for achieving inch loss around the abdomen. However, routines for the spine and the muscles at the back of the shoulders are included for a general improvement in the posture, which will generally improve appearance.

Each plan consists of a warm-up and cool-down phase. The exercises involve repeated movements designed to gradually strengthen different sets of muscles and it is suggested that the dieter will benefit most if the programme is performed every day. These exercises can easily be performed at home and can be used in conjunction with aerobic forms of exercise such as vigorous walking or cycling, which will improve general fitness.

Extras

To maintain a flat stomach after the programme has been completed it is suggested that the dieter continues to eat low-fat foods but increases the calorie intake gradually and, as a very occasional treat, enjoys some of the foods that would not be permitted on the diet plan. The ten tips in the maintenance section also include a recommendation for continuing with the exercise programme.

Full information about this diet is published in *Rosemary Conley's Complete Flat Stomach Plan* by Rosemary Conley (Arrow, 1996) £7.99.

The Food Combining Diet

THE Food Combining Diet is a 28-day weight loss programme developed from Dr Hay's theories on managing food combination in order to eliminate the build-up of toxins in the body. It does not involve calorie counting.

Recommended for
It is recommended for gradual weight loss and detoxification.

Not recommended for
It is not recommended for those whose priority is rapid weight loss or spot-reduction of specific areas of the body.

Advocates of food combining believe that the inadequate elimination of waste products from the body can occur when protein and starch are mixed within the same meal. The enzymes that digest proteins need an acid environment to act effectively, whereas the enzymes for breaking down starches need an alkaline environment. This results in incomplete digestion when these foods are combined in one meal, which ultimately results in poor absorption of nutrients and poor elimination of waste products.

There are five basic rules to the Food Combining Diet:
• Do not mix sugar or starchy foods with proteins within one meal
• Increase your intake of fresh fruits, vegetables and salads
• Always eat fruits in isolation; do not mix them with other foods
• Do not mix milk with protein or starch within one meal
• Avoid foods which are processed or refined

There are no forbidden foods on the diet but the recommended foods are generally low fat, fresh and natural.

To simplify the process of food combining the author has developed a system whereby foods can be identified as acid-forming or alkaline-forming or neutral, and a diet plan is produced that uses these foods in the right balance and in the right combination. The diet tends to be heavier in alkaline-forming foods (e.g. fresh fruits, vegetables and salads) with acid-forming foods, such as meat and fish, carefully combined to establish optimum nutrition.

The programme also includes a 24-hour Detox Diet using alkaline-forming foods only (fresh fruits and vegetables). This is designed to rest digestion and eliminate toxins from the bloodstream. Drinking plenty of fresh water and cutting down on caffeine and tea is emphasised at this stage, although it is recommended throughout the Food Combining Diet.

Menu Plans are provided for a four-week period providing three basic meals with snacks and desserts included on specific days. Each meal is clearly identified as either alkaline- or acid-forming, starch or protein based, enabling the dieter to become accustomed to the foods and their combinations.

A typical day's menu
Breakfast (starch):
Home-made muesli
Mid-morning snack (alkaline):
Small bunch of grapes
Lunch (alkaline):
Vegetable crudités with avocado dip
Evening meal (protein):
Grilled lemon sole with green salad

In addition to the four-week plan there are food lists which clearly show which specific foods can be combined for protein, starch and neutral meals and an at-a-glance reference chart to show the best combinations of food groups. The Food Combining Diet features meal suggestions which are appropriate for vegetarians. Many of the menu options do require some preparation. Until accustomed to food combining, the dieter might find it difficult to devise their own meals for packed lunches or when in a hurry.

Eating out
There are no specific recommendations for eating out and the dieter may feel that he or she needs to be experienced in food combining before being able to eat in a restaurant.

How fast is it?

There is no average weight loss rate on the Food Combining diet. Author Kathryn Marsden believes that in following the plan, weight will be lost at a steady, gradual rate and target weight will be permanently maintained.

Exercise

There is no specific exercise programme but the author recommends that 15 to 20 minutes exercise should be performed each day.

Extras

Using the four-week plan should enable the dieter to get to grips with the practice of food combining, which can then be developed as a lifestyle approach to eating.

The diet also looks at the importance of good blood circulation, for promoting the supply of nutrients to body cells and removing the waste products for elimination. If the body is suffering toxic overload then this system of delivery and removal slows down and the toxin levels rise even further. Exercise and skin brushing can help to improve the circulation and thereby promote the supply of nutrition and the lymphatic drainage of waste products.

Full information about this diet is published in *The Food Combining Diet* by Kathryn Marsden (Thorsons, 1993) £4.99.

Vegetarian Slimming

THE Vegetarian Slimming plan comprises three diet programmes based around vegetarian and vegan meals – a calorie-counted plan, a hip and thigh diet and a weight loss plan for food-combiners. It is recommended for vegetarians, vegans or anyone who wishes to lose weight on a meat-free programme. The diet features short-term quick diets for attaining rapid weight loss.

The Vegetarian Slimming Plan for Calorie-Counters

This diet is based on an intake of 1000 calories per day, with extra calories available from recommended Diet Boosters snacks. It is recommended that women with 14 lb (6.5 kg) or less to lose stick to a daily intake of 1000 calories. Women with more than 14 lb (6.5 kg) to lose should set their intake at 1200 per day, and women with more than 42 lb (19 kg) to lose should set their daily allowance at 1500 calories. Men are recommended to set their daily allowance at 1200 or 1500 calories, again depending upon the amount of weight they have to lose.

Each daily menu is devised for breakfast, lunch and an evening meal, with an additional 200 calorie allowance for pasteurised milk, or soya alternative, and fruit. The dieter can choose from recipe options for each meal (all of which have been calorie-counted) and those on a higher calorific intake can choose calorie-counted choices from the lists of Diet Boosters and Treats. A list of unlimited vegetables is also provided.

A typical day's menu
Breakfast
Scrambled egg on toast
Lunch
Beany salad
Evening Meal
Quick home-made pizza with salad

The Vegetarian Slimming Plan for Food Combiners

This is presented as an alternative weight-loss plan for those who do not like calorie-counting. Based on the principles of the Hay system, it aims to facilitate the loss of excess fat by establishing a more efficient digestive process. As with the Food Combining Diet, proteins and carbohydrates are eaten separately. A list of foods that should not be mixed is provided and the recipes are labelled as either carbohydrate or protein or neutral. Other advice includes eating at least one fruit-only meal a day, avoiding sugar and artificial sweeteners and leaving at least three hours between each meal.

The plan provides suggestions for breakfasts, lunches and evening meals, which include recipes such as Spiced Vegetables with Brown Rice and Sliced Onion and Tomato (carbohydrate), and Spinach Roulade with Peas and Carrots and Continental Leaf Salad (protein). Sample menus are provided to help the dieter become accustomed to the method of vegetarian food combining.

In addition to the individual diets the Vegetarian Slimming plan also provides over 100 calorie-counted recipes which are coded as follows; V = Vegan; HT = Hip and Thigh; FV = Fruit and Vegetable; N = Neutral; C = Carbohydrate; P = Protein. This enables the dieter to choose meals which will be appropriate to her chosen plan.

The Vegetarian Hip and Thigh Diet

Author Rose Elliot argues that a vegetarian diet, which has a high content of fresh fruit and vegetables and contains no saturated fat, is suited to shifting stubborn fat and diminishing cellulite on the hip and thigh area.

The dieter is instructed to begin this programme on a one-day Pineapple and Banana Diet, which consists of pineapple for breakfast, lunch and an evening meal, with two large bananas last thing at night and water, black tea and coffee or herbal tea to drink. After this the dieter can then move on to the Quick Fruit Cleansing Diet, for another two to three days, or the Rice and Fruit Diet for up to two weeks.

These diets are short-term measures for eliminating toxins and promoting rapid weight loss and are not to be adopted long term as they are are not nutritionally balanced. It is recommended that when on these diets you avoid alcohol, nicotine and coffee.

Once the dieter has completed this quick-start plan, she can then move on to choose three meals a day from the Food Combiners plan. The meals which are appropriate for the Hip and Thigh plan are clearly coded. It is recommended that breakfast is a fruit meal and that at least one other meal features fresh vegetables, for example a lunchtime salad. The recipes which are recommended for the Hip and Thigh plan are wheat-free and use limited amounts of cow's milk and dairy products. An example of the meals for the plan is as follows: citrus-marinated tofu with stir-fry vegetables, aubergines with soy and ginger and a piece of fresh fruit.

This plan is supplemented with advice on various techniques for diminishing cellulite, such as skin brushing, massage and exercise.

Eating out
General advice for eating out and entertaining while dieting are given. Rose Elliot points out that many of the vegetarian alternatives on pub and restaurant menus are often not ideal for a slimmer and she recommends that you are cautious when selecting options. Practical tips are given on how to save calories and minimise on the consumption of fats when in a restaurant.

How fast is it?
The average weight loss for a slimmer on the 1000 calorie-counted plan is estimated at around 2 lb (1 kg) a week. Variations will occur in the speed of weight loss, depending on the plan followed. On the short-term quick diets the weight loss will be more rapid, as the daily calorific intake is very low. On the Hip and Thigh and the Food Combining plans the rate of weight loss may be more gradual, since calorie restriction is not the primary concern.

Exercise
The Vegetarian Slimming plan provides simple stretching and toning exercises, along with a yoga routine, which Rose Elliot recommends for improving muscle tone and flexibility. However, the dieter is encouraged to take part in any form of physical activity that will be safe and enjoyable.

Extras
Rose Elliot provides general nutritional information on vegetarian foods, advising that if in doubt the dieter should take a vitamin B_{12} supplement. Various health, ethical and ecological issues relating to vegetarianism are also examined.

A section on meditation and relaxation addresses the emotional and psychological factors which are involved in gaining excess weight. Rose Elliot suggests that by using relaxation techniques the mind and body can work in harmony to establish sustained health and vitality.

Further information on this diet is published in *Vegetarian Slimming* by Rose Elliot (Orion, 1996) £5.99.

Rosemary Conley's
Complete Hip and Thigh Diet

THIS phenomenally commercially successful diet plan is a low-fat eating plan and exercise programme aimed at spot-reduction, primarily in the hip and thigh area, and also intended to achieve long-term weight loss.

Recommended for
It is recommended primarily for fat loss in the hip and thigh area. However, dieters who have used the programme have reported general weight and inch loss. The diet also emphasises the importance of learning new eating habits.

Not recommended for
It is not recommended for pregnant women and anyone with a diagnosed medical condition should not use the diet or the exercise plan.

The programme was originally devised after Rosemary Conley, a seasoned slimmer, was forced to go on a low-fat diet to avoid surgery for a gallstone problem. To her astonishment she found that in simply cutting down on fat she had managed to lose weight and, significantly, inches from her hips and thighs, areas which had steadfastly resisted her previous weight loss attempts.

Many pear-shaped women have experienced the frustration of following a strict calorie-controlled diet and losing weight, but not in the areas they feel most unhappy with. It is notoriously difficult to shift extra weight once it has accumulated on the hip and thigh area. However, Rosemary Conley believes that in combining a low-fat eating plan with an exercise programme it really is possible to permanently lose this fat.

How fast is it?
The average weight loss, cited by the author, is 2 lb (1 kg) a week. The

average overall inch loss for dieters who adhered to the programme for 10 weeks was 14.5 inches. A staggering 92 per cent of respondents reported that they achieved a significant inch loss in the hip and thigh area.

The diet plan is based on three meals a day: breakfast, lunch and a dinner menu, which includes three courses. The dieter is advised to avoid snacking through the day but it is possible to use one of the courses of the dinner option as a supper snack, if necessary. The eating plan is very flexible with a good selection for vegetarians and a plan for packed lunches.

There is a list of forbidden foods which includes fats and oils, full-fat milk, cream, fried food, meat products, crisps, chocolate, cakes, biscuits and egg yolks.

It is recommended that the dieter tries to select menus that will balance the following daily nutritional recommendations:

- 6 oz (150 g) protein food (fish, meat, poultry, cottage cheese and baked beans)
- 12 oz (300 g) vegetables
- 12 oz (300 g) fresh fruit (including fruit juice)
- 6 oz (150 g) carbohydrate (bread, cereals, potatoes, rice, pasta)
- 10 fl oz (250 ml) skimmed or semi-skimmed milk

The author also recommends that one multivitamin tablet should be taken each day, to ensure that the recommended daily vitamin intake is sustained.

All vegetables, including potatoes, can be eaten in unlimited quantities, as long as they are prepared and eaten without fat. Pasta can be eaten instead of rice, potatoes or a similar carbohydrate, as long as it is egg-free and does not contain fat. Red meat is restricted to two helpings a week. All yoghurts and cottage cheeses should be low-fat. If temptation strikes between meals, chopped celery, peppers, tomatoes or carrots can be used to fill the gap.

Breakfast can be chosen from one of three plans – cereal, cooked, and continental and fruit; lunch from one of four plans – fruit, packed, cold and hot, and dinner from starters, desserts, vegetarian and non-vegetarian main courses. There are over 150 recipes provided in addition to the meal suggestions included in each plan. None of the meals or recipes are calorie-counted and it is up to the dieter to make an individual selection from each menu programme.

A typical day's menu
Breakfast
5 oz (125 g) stewed fruit (no sugar) with 1 diet yoghurt
Lunch
Rice salad (chopped onion, peppers, tomatoes, peas sweetcorn and
    cucumber with boiled brown rice sprinkled with soy sauce)
Dinner
Starter – garlic mushrooms
Main course – steamed, grilled or microwaved trout, stuffed with prawns
    and served with a large salad or assorted vegetables
Dessert – sliced banana served with fresh raspberries or strawberries

A daily allowance is made for one alcoholic drink for women and two for men, 10 fl oz (250 ml) skimmed milk and 4 fl oz (100 ml) unsweetened fruit juice.

Eating out
Eating out is not specifically addressed by the Complete Hip and Thigh Diet. However, one of the aims of the programme is to encourage people to recognise the fat content of foods and to make permanent low-fat changes to their diet. Once a dieter is accustomed to this he or she may find that enjoying low-fat options in a restaurant is not too much of a problem.

Exercise
The importance of exercise for boosting the metabolism, burning off fat and improving muscle tone is emphasised by Rosemary Conley. The exercises follow a complete programme – warm-up routines; aerobic exercise for fitness and fat-burning; a series of body-shaping exercises for toning and strengthening muscles in the hip and thigh area and repetitive stretch exercises for a cool-down phase.

Extras
The author claims that because the calorie intake on the diet is relatively high (in comparison to other diets) then the problem of rebound weight

gain is diminished. Once the target weight is reached the low-fat plan can be adopted as the basis for permanent eating habits. In this way the dieter can stick to a low-fat eating plan and add more of the foods recommended on the diet.

The author also claims that by following the programme many women have experienced a significant cellulite loss. Other methods of treatment, such as massaging with creams, and using toning tables and passive exercise machines are analysed, leading the author to the conclusion that effective treatment of cellulite is best achieved by the combination of exercise and a healthy, low-fat diet.

Full information about this diet is published in *Rosemary Conley's Complete Hip and Thigh Diet* by Rosemary Conley (Arrow, 1993) £4.99.

Rosemary Conley's
Metabolism Booster Diet

ROSEMARY Conley's Metabolism Booster Diet uses the low-fat food philosophy that was so successful in her *Complete Hip and Thigh Diet*, and incorporates this into a complete series of diet plans and exercises designed to shed excess fat and boost the metabolism.

Recommended for
Achieving permanent weight loss and avoiding rebound weight gain. The diet takes a flexible approach that will cater for various lifestyles.

Not recommended for
Dieters aiming specifically at spot-reduction. The author advises that anyone planning to embark on a weight loss programme should first consult their GP.

The author of the diet claims that the key to successful and permanent weight loss lies in increasing the metabolic rate. This can be achieved by combining exercise with an eating plan which allows a higher calorific intake than most diets. This resolves the problem of rebound weight gain which occurs when the body readjusts the basal metabolic rate in response to continued calorie restriction.

The emphasis on a low-fat approach stems from evidence which suggests that such a diet may facilitate greater weight loss than a non low-fat diet of exactly the same calorific value. Thus by concentrating on significantly reducing the fat content of a diet the actual calorific content may not need to be restricted to a degree whereby the body responds with an automatic lowering of the basal metabolic rate.

The programme has been devised to enable the dieter to choose a plan that will fit in with his or her lifestyle. This also enables the slimmer to establish eating habits and patterns that can be comfortably continued once the desired amount of weight has been lost.

The lifestyle diet options
- Six Meals-a-Day Plan
- Freedom Diet
- Four Meals-a-Day Diet
- Eat Yourself Slim Diet
- Three Two-Course Meals-a-Day Diet
- Gourmet Diet
- Vegetarian Diet
- Lazy Cook's Diet

In addition to these diets, there are Seasonal Menu Plans which provide low-fat alternatives for entertaining at those difficult times of the year when food is an important part of celebration and socialising.

Each of the plans has been devised for a 30-day period, with full daily menus and recipes which can be followed without having to count calories or even fat units. The range of the diet plans should cater for every lifestyle and preference. For example, the Six Meals-a-Day Plan is ideal for those who tend to be great 'pickers' and prefer the 'little and often' approach, whereas the Gourmet Diet should satisfy the adventurous and enthusiastic cook. In contrast the Lazy Cook's Diet, with its recommendations for healthy low-fat convenience foods, is ideal for anyone with a very busy lifestyle or an abhorrence of cooking.

With the emphasis firmly on flexibility and enjoyment, the dieter can choose to substitute meals in relation to personal preference. For example, should the evening meal suggestion for Day 5 not appeal then the evening meal from any of the other 29 days can be substituted. However, whilst on one plan it is important not to use recipes or suggestions from any other plan, since each programme has been nutritionally devised in accordance with the number of meals and courses presented.

The 'forbidden foods' include all fats and oils, high-fat dairy products, many meat products, chocolates, cakes and biscuits, cocoa and high-fat fruits and vegetables, such as avocado.

The recommended nutritional balance for each diet plan (which is the same as the balance for the *Complete Hip and Thigh Diet*) provides the basis for a range of highly imaginative and versatile recipes which will delight even the most seasoned dieter.

A typical day's menu
Breakfast
Home-made muesli
Lunch
Jacket potato with ratatouille
Evening Meal
Tomato and pepper soup
Steak surprise or vegetable bake
Fruit sorbet

How fast is it?
The average weight loss should be around 2 lb (1 kg) per week, depending on how much exercise is combined with the eating plan.

Exercise
Of course, boosting the metabolism involves a certain commitment to physical activity. The form of exercise advocated by this diet programme is low-impact aerobics, which can be performed either in an appropriate class or in the home according to the recommended instructions. Anybody planning to begin the exercise programme is advised to refer to a pulse rate chart. This will enable each individual to define a basic activity rate at which exercise can be performed to a beneficial and safe level. It is recommended that at least 15 minutes of exercise is performed three times a week.

Extras
Once the dieter has reached his or her personal goal of weight/fat loss, a maintenance programme can be used to ensure that all the good dieting work is sustained. This does not involve following a prescriptive plan for a 'transition' phase; the emphasis is placed on continuing to follow a low-fat approach to eating and avoiding or moderating certain foods. Similarly, a continuation of exercise is recommended to boost the metabolism and to support general health, and advice is given here for pacing physical activity appropriately.

Full information about this diet is published in *Rosemary Conley's Metabolism Booster Diet* by Rosemary Conley (Arrow, 1992) £4.99.

The LifePoints Diet

THE LifePoints Diet is a comprehensive programme, aimed at long-term, gradual weight loss, which overhauls methods for counting calories or fat units in favour of a new approach – assessing and using foods in terms of their LifePoints or RiskPoints.

Recommended for
Permanent weight loss and maximising health and vitality.

Not recommended for
Anyone whose priority is fast weight loss.

The diet places emphasis on the importance of maintaining a balanced eating plan which allows the dieter to enjoy all the vital nutrients. Foods are assessed in terms of a score for their healthy components (LifePoints) or their unhealthy components (RiskPoints). It is recommended that the dieter aims for a daily intake of at least 100 LifePoints and, initially, no more than 75 RiskPoints (a total that can be readjusted to a higher value of up to 125 once satisfactory weight loss has been achieved). To achieve an adequate nutritional balance, foods should be chosen from four specified food groups:
- Fruit and Fruit Juices
- Cereals, Grains and Pasta
- Vegetables and Vegetable Products and Legumes
- Nuts and Seeds

Foods from a further two categories – Meat, Fish and Dairy; and Drinks, Desserts, Snacks and Sauces – are optional.

In this way the diet can be used as a flexible tool for weight loss and for then establishing a healthy approach to eating in the long term.

To begin the diet it is recommended that the dieter uses the Kick-start plan, a seven-day programme which will enable the slimmer to become accustomed to the LifePoints approach by using daily menu plans for breakfast, lunch, dinner and two snacks.

A typical day's menu from the Kick-start plan
Breakfast (LifePoints = 54/RiskPoints = 15)
Grape nuts cereal with skimmed milk
Half a cantaloupe melon
1 glass of fresh, unsweetened orange juice
1 cup of tea or coffee with milk
Morning Snack (LifePoints = 27/RiskPoints = 0)
1 carrot and 1 stick of celery cut into sticks with
3 oz (90 g) of Bean Pâté (according to recipe)
1 glass of tomato juice
Lunch (LifePoints = 41/RiskPoints = 20)
1 vegetable burger served in a bun with a mixed vegetable salad and low-
    fat French dressing
1 glass of pineapple juice
1 bowl of fresh raspberries or blackberries with a crispbread or a rice
    cake
Afternoon Snack (LifePoints = 20/RiskPoints = 2)
1 handful of dried figs
1 glass of carrot juice
Dinner (LifePoints = 111/RiskPoints = 19)
Cream of Mushroom Soup
Marinated Steak and Mushrooms with Roast Potatoes
Steamed chicory greens and steamed carrots
Fresh raspberries or blackberries
Daily Total = 253 LifePoints/46 RiskPoints

After using the Kick-start plan the dieter will be able to go solo, using food
charts (calculated to LifePoints and RiskPoints values) to establish an
individual daily eating plan, with the added insurance of over 40 varied
and imaginative recipes to fall back on. There is plenty of scope for packed
lunches and the plan is entirely appropriate for vegetarians.

Each food's value is calculated according to weight or size, so portion
control is an important consideration in making the diet work effectively.
However, the in-built flexibility of this approach means that a food which
is relatively high in RiskPoints, such as a snack bar of chocolate or a
doughnut, can be incorporated into the diet on a particular day if the
intake for the rest of that day is then controlled to ensure that the RiskPoints
do not exceed their limit.

Eating out

While there is no specific advice for eating out, the dieter will find that the comprehensive list of LifePoints foods can be used to cope with figuring out the most appropriate options on a restaurant menu.

How fast is it?

The LifePoints Diet aims for easy, enjoyable weight loss without traditional restriction or the risk of hunger pangs. The rate of weight loss will, therefore, be gradual. However, this is balanced in that the diet does aim for permanent weight loss and a long-term re-education of dietary habit.

Exercise

The authors of the LifePoints Diet emphasise the value of exercise for maximising weight loss and vitality. The Kick-start plan includes a series of repetitive stretch exercises designed to improve suppleness and strength, which can be performed at home or even in the office. The dieter is invited to choose six of these exercises and perform them daily for a few weeks.

A walking programme has been devised to allow the individual to gradually develop a general level of fitness, which can then be extended to a more specific form of exercise. Recommendations are made for taking part in aerobic and anaerobic activity, such as swimming, cycling and yoga, along with sensible advice on how to enjoy the benefits of exercising without risking injury or illness. The general health benefits of physical activity are also fully analysed.

Extras

The diet also includes a comprehensive analysis of vitamins and minerals and advice on how to maximise nutritional benefits from food through ensuring its freshness and using the best preparation and cooking techniques. Questionnaires and charts enable dieters to become more accustomed to the whole issue of nutrition and their individual approach to eating. In addition to this, handy dietary tips and facts are dotted throughout the book, reinforcing the philosophy that the diet can be used as a programme for weight loss and as a lifestyle guide for healthy eating.

Full information about this diet is published in *LifePoints Diet* by Peter Cox and Peggy Brusseau (Bloomsbury, 1996) £4.99.

The Complete F-Plan Diet

THE F-Plan Diet has now been around for over a decade and is essentially a high-fibre, low-fat, calorie-controlled weight loss plan. However, despite the benefits, some dieters have found that increasing dietary fibre can initially be accompanied by an increase in flatulence. This should subside once the body gets used to its new high-fibre intake.

Recommended for
It is recommended for general weight loss without hunger and for establishing long-term habits for healthy eating.

Not recommended for
It is not recommended if you if you suffer from certain bowel or stomach disorders and have been instructed by your doctor to avoid certain types of fibre.

In recent years the importance of including dietary fibre in our diets has been supported by much medical research. It is recommended that we eat at least 30 g of fibre each day – in the UK, however, the average daily intake is approximately only 20 g.

Advantages to maintaining a high-fibre diet:
- Many high-fibre foods are low in fat, and fibre that is derived from cereals reduces the absorption of cholesterol.
- Conditions of the lower digestive system, such as constipation, diverticulitis and haemorrhoids, have been linked to diets that are low in fibre content. Increasingly high-fibre diets are being used in the prevention and treatment of such conditions.
- Carbohydrates from fibre-rich foods are released more slowly than carbohydrates derived from refined, processed foods. This can be regarded as beneficial in the prevention of maturity-onset diabetes, a form of the condition associated with obesity and a poor diet.

Naturally the dieter stands to gain from these health benefits; however, the author claims that using high-fibre foods in a calorie-controlled diet has specific advantages for anyone attempting to lose weight.

How a high-fibre diet helps weight loss:

- Fibre-rich foods tend to be more filling (staying in the stomach for longer) and the dieter will feel more satisfied, reducing the risk of breaking the diet through hunger.
- Fibre is not digested by the body and therefore a proportion of the calories eaten during the day will not be stored by the body. These will be expelled in the faeces and promote a more rapid rate of weight loss.
- Following a high-fibre diet for the purposes of weight reduction should enable the individual to establish a healthier way of eating. This is particularly valuable if the dieter is to avoid regaining some of the lost weight, once the diet has ended.

The F-Plan Diet recommends a daily calorific intake of 1000 to 1250 calories for women and around 1500 calories for men. The recommended fibre intake is at least 30 g per day.

Some people may regard high-fibre food as a rather daunting (if not unpalatable) combination of cereal bran, vegetables and fruit. However, the meals and recipes included in the F-Plan Diet are designed to combine fibre with fish, low-fat dairy products, eggs, poultry and lean meat. This ensures that a balance of proteins, essential fats, calcium, vitamins and minerals is maintained, and has the additional benefit of enabling the dieter to eat a varied, appetising menu.

Typical high-fibre foods used in the F-Plan diet include wholewheat pasta and bread, baked beans, kidney beans, baked potatoes, lentils, sweetcorn, salad vegetables and dried and fresh fruit.

There are six eating plans included in the diet which have been designed to cater for individual needs:
- Simply F-Plan
- F-Plan for Working Women
- Keen Cook's F-Plan
- Canned and Packaged F-Plan
- F-Plan for Men
- F-Plan for Children

It is recommended that one portion of Fibre-filler is included in each day's intake. This is a mixture of high-fibre breakfast cereals, nuts and dried fruits which provides 200 calories and 15 g of fibre. (The recipe for the Fibre-filler can be found in The Complete F-Plan Diet).

A typical day's menu from the F-Plan for Working Women

Daily allowance
1 portion of Fibre-filler
$^1/_2$ pint (285 ml) skimmed milk
1 orange, apple or pear

Breakfast
Half a portion of the Fibre-filler served with half the daily milk allowance

Lunch
10.6 oz (300 g) can Heinz Lentil Soup
2 Energen F-Plan Brancrisps, lightly spread with Marmite or yeast extract
1 orange

Evening Meal
Watercress and herb omelette
4 oz (115 g) fresh or frozen peas
1 $7^3/_4$ oz (220 g) can Boots Shapers Peaches in Low-cal Syrup for dessert

Supper
Remainder of the Fibre-filler served with milk from the daily allowance
An apple or pear from the daily allowance.

A variety of low-calorie, high-fibre recipes are provided for main meals and meal suggestions are made for sandwiches, soups, pastas, baked potatoes, salads and desserts. All of these are calculated in terms of their calorific and fibre totals. The F-Plan Diet is appropriate for vegetarians and the eating plans are easy to follow.

Eating out
The problem of business lunches and socialising in restaurants is addressed in the F-Plan Diet. The basic advice given is for the dieter to use common sense and to stick to relatively simple dishes.

How fast is it?
The author of the F-Plan Diet claims that the average weight loss is 3 lb (1.4 kg) per week. The dieter is encouraged to adopt aspects of the diet

(for example, using wholewheat pasta and bread and eating fresh fruits and vegetables) on a permanent basis in order to maintain healthy eating habits.

Exercise
There is no specific exercise programme with the F-Plan Diet.

Extras
Charts of basic and prepackaged foods, calculated for calorie and fibre content, are provided.

Full information about this diet is published in *The Complete F-Plan Diet* by Audrey Eyton (Penguin Books, 1988) £6.99.

Dean Ornish's Life Choice, Eat More, Weigh Less Diet

DR Dean Ornish, a specialist in cardiac disease, was interested in the part played by diet in controlling heart and circulatory illness in severely affected patients. He devised a low-fat, mainly vegetarian diet for his heart patients, which often involved them eating greater quantities, but of different types of food, than they had consumed previously. As well as having a beneficial effect on the health of the heart, it was noted that patients routinely lost weight while following the diet. This plan is built upon obtaining no more than 10 per cent of daily calories from fat and never eating food that contains more than 2 g of fat per serving.

Recommended for
Those who need to lose weight because they suffer from or are at risk of heart disease.

Not recommended for
Growing children who need essential fats in their diet.

A wide variety of recipes are provided, based upon whole grains, peas, beans and pulses, vegetables and fruit. Other foods, permitted in small amounts, include very low-fat or no-fat dairy products and some commercially-prepared foods, as long as these are also low in sugar content. Foods to be avoided are all those that contain 2 g of fat per serving, meat, poultry, fish, oils, margarines, dairy produce, nuts, seeds, sugar and alcohol. Dean Ornish's recipes are tasty, nutritious and satisfying but may contain ingredients which are not readily available in all parts of the British Isles so some adaptations may be necessary.

A typical day's menu
Breakfast
Portion of cantaloupe or other melon

Fat-free cottage cheese
Spicy persimmon muffin
Sugar-free fruit preserve
Hot drink with fat-free milk
Lunch
Wholewheat burito filled with a portion of whole grain rice, mixed with
    beans and vegetables
Green side salad
Portion of sugar and fat-free chutney or dressing
Dinner
Lentil soup with garlic croutons
Spinach ravioli
Green side salad
Fruit

This diet has proved successful both in helping people to lose weight and
in protecting the health of the heart, with the added benefit of allowing a
good quantity of certain foods to be eaten, so preventing hunger pangs.
The diet is even more successful when accompanied by a regular
programme of exercise. Dr Ornish has devised two main diet programmes,
both primarily aimed at protecting the heart but with the 'side effect' of
weight loss. These are 'The Reversal Diet' for people who already have
diagnosed cardiac disease and 'The Prevention Diet', for those who have
a cholesterol level of 150 or less and who wish to protect their heart.

Further details can be obtained from the book, *Dean Ornish's Life Choice,
Eat More, Weight Less Diet* by Dean Ornish, MD, (HarperCollins, 1993).

Several other diet plans follow similar guidelines to those of Dean Ornish,
including those of Dr Terry Shintani, Dr John McDougall and Dr Gabe
Mirkin. These diets drastically reduce the amount of fat that is eaten and
base their weight loss programme upon the consumption of beans, whole
grains, vegetables and fruits, with some low-fat dairy products allowed
and other foods included only rarely or not at all.

The Pritikin Diet

THE Pritikin Diet was developed by Nathan Pritikin about ten years before that of Dr Dean Ornish. It is an extremely low-fat diet, in which only 10 per cent of calories are derived from fat with the rest being obtained from complex, unrefined carbohydrate such as vegetables, peas and beans, whole grains and fruits. Low-fat animal protein and fat-free dairy produce such as skimmed milk is permitted in very small amounts and daily exercise is recommended. The diet was primarily developed as a means of preventing heart disease but weight loss is achieved by nearly all those who embark upon the Pritikin programme which seeks to help people to permanently change to a healthier lifestyle.

Recommended for
Those who need to lose weight because they suffer from or are at risk of heart disease.

Not recommended for
Growing children who need essential fats in their diet.

A typical day's menu:
Breakfast
Wholewheat, high-fibre, low-fat cereal or porridge with skimmed milk
Grapefruit
Lunch
Wholewheat pitta bread with green salad and raw vegetables, fat-free dressing, if desired
1 small bowl of lentil soup
Dinner
Vegetable soup
Wholegrain rice and bean salad
Steamed vegetables (broccoli, courgettes)
Slice of rye bread
Stewed apple and fat-free yoghurt

Some concerns have been raised that the diets are too low in fat, if adopted permanently and that a lack of dietary fatty acids may lead to inadequate absorption of vitamins and minerals. However, both the Pritikin diet and the Dean Ornish diet have been shown to be effective in treating cardiovascular disease, lowering blood cholesterol and promoting weight loss.

Nathan Pritikin's books contain recipes and cooking instructions which show readers how to prepare a variety of tasty and satisfying meals. However, some western people find it hard to adhere to the diet on a permanent basis since it involves giving up most of the foods which they hold dear! Once weight loss has been achieved, a helpful approach might be to adopt the Pritikin or Ornish diet programme as a basis and not to worry too much about the occasional lapse, as long as there is no complete return to former patterns of eating.

The Pritikin diet plans are outlined in several books including *The Pritikin Permanent Weight-Loss Manual* and *The Pritikin Programme for Diet and Exercise* (Bantam Doubleday Dell Publishing, £9.40).

The Glucose Revolution

THE *Glucose Revolution* is not a diet plan as such, but a guide to healthy eating employing the theory of the glycemic index (GI) as "a scientifically validated tool for the dietary management of diabetes, heart disease, weight loss and athletic performance" and has detailed sections on each aspect. The authors say that their work is a "revolution" because it will change the way that people approach health and weight loss and the way they eat. They claim it is an easier and more effective method of losing weight than any other.

Recommended for

Because this book does not advocate eating less or cutting down on calories, and promotes a healthy, wholefood, nutritionally-balanced diet, this diet is suitable for everyone.

It is claimed that those who follow the diet may be less likely to develop diabetes and heart disease. It is claimed that low GI diets can help control established diabetes, can help people lose weight, may help lower blood lipids and can improve the body's sensitivity to insulin.

It has the additional benefit, for those for whom other low-fat diets have proved unsuccessful, of providing a diet that avoids tedious calorie counting, hunger pangs, cravings and crankiness.

The glycemic index is a rating system indicating how different foods affect levels of blood sugar. Foods with a low GI promote a slow rise in blood sugar which keeps hunger at bay and encourages the body to dissolve body fat by converting it into energy.

After you eat, the level of glucose rises in the blood. Some foods (those with a high GI) make blood sugar rise faster. Eating these kinds of foods has a number of knock-on effects. A rapid and high rise in blood sugar corresponds to a high rise in the production of insulin. High insulin levels stimulate the appetite causing you to want to eat more, probably of the same type of high GI snacks thus creating a vicious circle. When insulin levels are high, fewer calories are burned. The rush in insulin causes a rapid dip in blood sugar levels. In response to this the body produces adrenaline which causes edginess, irritability, poor concentration and fatigue. This is a reason why bingeing on snacks such as chips and cookies is the worst thing you can do if you are feeling stressed as it exacerbates the symptoms.

The Glucose Revolution diet is a low-fat, high-carbohydrate diet (in the form of slow-release carbohydrate and whole grains) and includes lots of green vegetables and fruit, and some lean meat and fish.

Sugar is not necessarily forbidden. Sucrose (ordinary white sugar) has a GI of 67 while glucose (often found in sweets and candies) has a GI of 100. Sucrose is of only moderate GI Cornflakes have a GI of 84!

This book also gives recommendations of how much carbohydrate should be consumed by people of different sizes and lifestyles. The Western diet contains far too much food that is high in saturated fat and quick-release carbohydrate. Potatoes, white bread and some breakfast cereals, common elements in the diet of most Westerners, all have high GIs.

Relatively high GI foods include: those mentioned above as well as, bran flakes, brown bread (only wholegrain stoneground has a low GI), dates, french fries, rice cakes, waffles.

Relatively low GI foods include: apple juice, most fruits, oatmeal, pasta, muesli, butter beans, basmati rice, rye bread, yoghurt.

This book contains detailed but extremely readable and sensible explanations regarding nutrition.

A typical day's menu

The Glucose Revolution does not include detailed meal plans, but its easy-to-follow general nutritional information and guidance, recipes, and a listing of the GI values of common foods should provide you with more than enough information. However, it does contain a few menu examples such as the following:

Breakfast
All Bran or muesli
A poached egg on pumpernickel toast spread with a little butter
Lunch
A stoneground wheat roll with a light scraping of butter and a filling of chicken and salad

Home made vegetable soup
A piece of fruit
Dinner
High-carbohydrate grains or root vegetanbles
As many green vegetables as you like
A small amount of meat or, if you prefer, beans, lentils or tofu
Stewed fruit or a fruit sorbet
Snack ideas
2 portions of dairy produce (like a low fat yoghurt or a piece of cheese)
A slice of wholegrain toast
Half a bagel
Fruit
Vegetable sticks
Low-fat crackers and light cream cheese

Eating out
Although there is no specific information about eating out, the aim of *The Glucose Revolution* is to show you that as long as you are aware of the physiological effects of the food you are eating, and what you must do to counter those effects (such as consuming more low GI foods to counteract a high GI element in a meal), then no food is totally forbidden.

Exercise
Exercise is encouraged, but there is no specific exercise plan for weight loss outlined. However, there is a whole section on using the theory of the glycemic index to promote peak athletic performance.

Extras
Information on the latest nutritional research is included. And there are some tempting recipes and a listing of the GI values of foods. There are sections on heart disease, maintenance of diabetes, and athletic performance.

The Glucose Revolution is written by Jennie-Brand Miller, Ph.D.; Thomas M.S. Wolever M.D., Ph.D.; Stephen Colaguiri M.D. and Kaye Foster-Powell, M. Nutr. & Diet (first published as *The GI Factor* in 1996 in Australia by Hodder Headline Australia Pty Limited; published in the UK by Hodder Headline, 2000, UK; published in the USA by Marlowe & Company, 1999).

The G-Index Diet

THE *G-Index Diet* is one of several books on the market that encourage the incorporation of the scientifically-proven theory of the glycemic index (GI) into diet for weight loss. The theory has also been expounded for use by athletes, diabetics and patients with, or at risk of, heart disease. See also *The Glucose Revolution* by Jennie Brand-Miller et al (Hodder Headline, 2000) mentioned in the previous chapter and the *Schwarzbein Principle* by Dr Diana Schwarzbein (Marlowe and Company, 1999).

Recommended for

The diet is recommended for anyone because it emphasises the importance of regulating the blood sugar in a balanced, healthy diet rather than drastically reducing calorie intake. It may even increase the calorific intake of people who have been on traditional low-fat, high carbohydrate diets.

It is especially recommended if you have experienced irritability and anxiety through dieting, if you are making the transition from a low calorie liquid diet (usually for those who have 50 lbs or more to lose) back to a normal diet, and those who have dieted successfully up to a point but can't shift those last few pounds.

High GI foods actually increase your hunger. Some examples of these are: honey, baked potatoes, watermelon, carrots (in quantity), raisins, white bread, pastry, cornflakes, Shredded Wheat.

Low GI foods reduce the tendency to overeat. Some examples of these are: coarse wholegrain bread, pitta bread, wholemeal pasta, honeydew melon, green peppers, oatmeal, All Bran.

The diet is consistent with a low-fat, low-cholesterol, high-fibre diet. It encourages the consumption of:
* specially selected sugars and carbohydrates (low GI)
* strategic amounts of fat eaten at specific times to avoid cravings
* high amounts of fibre.

It provides a low-to-moderate calorie intake and there are no 'forbidden' foods.

The writer successfully lost 25lbs in three months on the regime and claims that he succesfully treats hundreds of his patients with the diet.

A typical day's menu

Breakfast
Porridge or All Bran or wholegrain toast and low-fat spread and 1 slice of trimmed drained bacon
A sliced pear
A sugar-free, non-fat yoghurt
Orange juice
Coffee

Lunch
Turkey sandwich on stoneground wholegrain bread with reduced-calorie mayonnaise or Pasta, bean and chickpea salad with low-calorie dressing
Skimmed milk

Dinner
Green salad with low-calorie dressing
Grilled chicken breast; boiled potato; broccoli
Strawberries
1 small square of chocolate, or 1 small piece of cheese, or a sugar-free, low-fat yoghurt

Snacks
Toasted pitta bread or a high-fibre muffin or a small square of cheddar cheese
3 tangerines
Sugar-free, non-fat yoghurt
Orange juice

Eating out
The author gives example of different kinds of restaurants and the best choices to make to maintain your low GI diet. He also gives a 14-day, detailed, calorie-counted eating-out plan for people who eat out frequently out of necessity.

How fast is it?
You can expect to lose approximately 1 to 2 lbs per week.

Exercise
There is no specific exercise programme with the G-Index Diet, although aerobic exercise is recommended.

Extras
The book includes recipes and a 21-day diet plan. There is also a GI food exchange list and hints on how to smoothly incorporate the theory into your life and develop flexibility in your approach to the diet. There is a detailed list of snacks and an explanation of when and why you should include them in your eating plan

The G-Index Diet by Richard N Podell, MD, FACP and William Proctor, (Warner Books, New York, 1993).

Weight Watchers

WEIGHT Watchers is a slimming club that combines a calorie-controlled eating programme with weekly classes. The organisation currently runs approximately 3700 classes throughout the UK, but also runs a postal scheme for dieters who cannot commit themselves to attending classes.

Recommended for

It is recommended for people who find it easier if they have supervision, support and advice in determining a successful weight-loss programme and establishing permanent, healthy eating habits. However, Weight Watchers require written approval from a GP before they will accept as members anyone who is pregnant, has a medical condition for which they are receiving treatment, or is aged under 10. They will not accept anyone suffering from an eating disorder or anyone who is less than 10 lb (4.5 kg) above the lowest recommended weight for their height.

Weight Watchers have devised their own diet plan which can be varied according to your age, gender and how much weight you have to lose. The aim of the programme is to promote a gradual weight loss while establishing a good dietary balance, which reflects the following guidelines:
- A balanced intake of a variety of foods
- Reduction in fat consumption
- Reduction in salt consumption
- Increase in the consumption of dietary fibre
- Reduction in the consumption of sugar

On joining Weight Watchers the dieter is weighed in private and a target weight and a diet plan agreed upon in consultation with a group leader. The dieter is then issued with introductory material and a menu plan for one week. This plan provides meal suggestions and recipe options for a breakfast, a light meal and a main meal, along with a daily allowance for low-fat milk and low-fat yoghurt.

After the first week the dieter can then stick to the menu plans which are supplied at the class each week. Alternatively, she can choose to create her own meal options in line with a selection system based on a daily balance of foods derived from the six nutritional groups below:

- 4 carbohydrate
- 3 fat
- 3 fruit
- 2 milk
- 5 protein
- 3 vegetable

On the selection system, specific foods and portions are listed to allow the dieter to easily calculate the appropriate intake and to swap equivalents. For example, if one recipe suggestion features rice, the dieter can substitute another carbohydrate (e.g. potato), if preferred. This flexible approach not only adds to the slimmer's satisfaction but also has great benefit in helping her to understand more about nutrition. However, portion control is very important in using the selection system since all the 'swaps' have been specifically calculated for nutritional value by weight. The dieter will then continue on this diet plan until target weight has been reached.

A typical day's menu
Breakfast
$1/2$ medium grapefruit
1 oz (30 g) cheese melted on 1 oz (30 g) slice of toast
Lunch
8 oz (240 g) baked potato
2 oz (60 g) cottage cheese or low-fat soft cheese with chopped chives
    and served with a mixed salad and 4 tablespoons of low-fat mayonnaise
1 pear
Dinner
3 oz (90 g) grilled pork or lamb chop or steak
8 oz (240 g) potato with 2 teaspoons of low-fat spread
carrots and cabbage
5 fl oz (150 ml) low-fat yoghurt

The Weight Watchers system also features recipes and plans for vegetarians.

Eating out
General advice for eating out will be given as part of the programme and can, of course, be discussed at group meetings.

Weight Watchers believe that it is important that their members do not feel deprived while on the programme and so they encourage a common sense approach to eating in restaurants and recommend light food during the day, prior to going out for a meal.

How fast is it?
The average weight loss is 1 to 2 lbs (0.5 to 1 kg) per week, although in the first two weeks weight loss may be more rapid.

Exercise
Exercise is recommended by Weight Watchers and general advice is given on aerobic, toning and stretching exercises. There are no exercise sessions involved with any of the classes – it is up to the dieter whether or not she wishes to supplement the eating plan with exercise. An aerobic work-out video is available from the organisation, for a fee.

Extras
A discussion session at Weight Watchers classes enables members to raise queries and address particular problems of dieting. Dieters can share their experiences with other members or speak to the group leader on an individual basis.

The group leader will monitor the progress of each dieter, offering advice and support as needed, and there are frequently demonstrations of recipes included in the diet plan.

Weight Watchers has a special maintenance programme which can be followed once target weight has been reached. This will involve gradually increasing calorie intake by choosing to add foods from the selection list.

It is possible to become a member of Weight Watchers even if you cannot attend the weekly classes since the diet plan is available on a postal scheme and you can also join online at www.weightwatchers.com. From this web address you can access Weight Watchers websites and classes all over the world.

There are numerous Weight Watcher's publications which can be viewed at an online bookshop such as Amazon.

Raw Foods Diets

AS the name suggests, followers of this dietary regime eat only raw foods which are inevitably plant-based – primarily whole grains, seeds, nuts, vegetables and fruits. People who go on a raw foods diet almost invariably lose weight. The foods are high in fibre and it requires effort and time to chew and eat them so fewer calories are taken in. Also, the foods themselves, apart from nuts and seeds, are low in calories and fat. Eating raw foods is good for health and digestion since valuable elements such as vitamins and minerals can be lost or destroyed through cooking. Raw fruit and vegetables provide valuable, low-calorie snacks for many people on weight-loss diets. However, most people find it very difficult to eat a raw foods diet alone or to follow it for any length of time.

From the point of view of healthy eating and weight reduction, it is unnecessary to adhere to a raw foods diet and, indeed, the benefits of doing so are open to question. This is because by insisting on raw foods alone, many helpful foods such as pulses and fish are excluded. Also, some health professionals have raised concerns about the safety of eating both intensively-produced and organic produce in a raw state. There is concern about the level of pesticides/chemicals in the former and pathogenic organisms in the latter. Thorough washing in cold, running water is recommended with removal of any part of the produce that appears to be damaged or diseased. Foods that require no cooking fit in well with busy lifestyles. They may be less suitable for those who like to eat three meals a day as it can be difficult to devise varied menus.

This type of diet is ideal for someone who likes to eat a little and often and who has a preference for these foods. There is little danger of over-eating but has the side effect of causing flatulence!

A raw foods diet should probably be viewed as a short-term option although some people remain on it for months, or even years. As mentioned above, including raw vegetables, fruits, nuts, seeds and grains into any diet, whether one is trying to lose weight or not, is very much a part of healthy eating. Information about raw foods diets is widely available in books, magazines and on the Internet.

The Fat Burner Diet

ON the Fat Burner Diet, the traditional approach to calculating foods purely in terms of their calorie content is rejected in favour of analysing foods for their complete nutritional balance and their effect upon the body. The authors believe that establishing a diet with a complete nutritional balance will burn off excess fat more efficiently.

Recommended for
Gradual, healthy weight loss – in supplying the body with a complete nutritional balance, the dieter is less likely to experience hunger and cravings and will enjoy maximum vitality.

Not recommended for
Spot reduction or rapid weight loss.

Based around weekly menu plans which provide three meals a day and snacks, the diet is essentially high in complex carbohydrates and fibre and low in fats and sugars. An emphasis is placed on eating proteins from low-fat and vegetarian sources, such as soya products, pulses and legumes.

The diet has been devised to reduce the intake of saturated fats and ensure an adequate intake of essential fatty acids (EFAs) which can be beneficial for conditions such as eczema, arthritis and asthma. A dietary intake which is low in saturated fats and provides EFAs will actually help to burn fat. Fish and seeds are good sources of EFAs.

The suitability of carbohydrates within the Fat Burner Diet depends on their complexity. Beans, lentils, wholegrains and vegetables are considered essential, with some fruits also valued within the dietary framework.

No sugar is permitted as, nutritionally, it is the emptiest of all foods and is easily converted to fat. Maintaining the stability of blood sugar levels is vital in the success of the programme. It is the level of glucose in the blood that determines appetite. When the level is low we feel hungry and may then be prone to overeating; when it is too high, the excess glucose is turned into glycogen, in the short term, and eventually into fat. It is recommended that sugar and sweet foods should be avoided altogether. However, different fruits have different effects on the blood-sugar levels, and bananas and dried fruit (which are considered weight-loss friendly in many other diets) are regarded as blood sugar agitators.

Avoid stimulants, such as caffeine, alcohol and nicotine. They stimulate the release of adrenaline which causes the body to react as if in response to a stressful situation. This raises blood sugar levels which then results in a release of insulin to tackle the raised glucose. This taxes the body so much that it can occasionally lead to the development of diabetes. All stimulants and aggravating food should be avoided in favour of foods that will calm the blood sugar levels.

Fibre is considered important as it helps protect against bowel cancer, diabetes and diverticular disease. Indigestible in the human gut, fibre satisfies hunger as it absorbs water and becomes bulkier in the digestive tract. The diet especially recommends konjac fibre (otherwise known as glucomannan). It can swell up to 100 times its volume and is excellent in the battle against weight gain, constipation and diabetes.

Vitamins are also considered vital for promoting health and vitality. The enzymes that help in the process of turning food into energy are dependent on a balance of eight vitamins and five nutrients. When there is a shortfall in any of these, food absorption does not occur efficiently and vitality is diminished. A balanced intake of vitamins is established by the diet to ensure that the metabolism is working at an optimum level.

Favoured foods on the diet include: vegetables, fruits, pulses, low-fat soya products, white fish, wholegrains, oats and rice cakes. Foods that are limited include dried fruit, nuts, bread, oily fish, low-fat cheese, eggs, tea and coffee. Foods such as high-fat meats and dairy products and sweets should be avoided altogether.

Along with the menu plans the Fat Burner Diet features delicious and varied recipes that reflect the careful nutritional plan.

A typical day's menu is as follows:
Breakfast
Fruit cocktail

Lunch
Nutty three bean salad

Dinner
Cheese and leek macaroni with green salad
Fruit fool
Snacks
Two pieces of fruit
Drinks
Unlimited water, herbal teas

Eating out
As with most weight-loss programmes, it is recommended that the diet plan is adhered to as strictly as possible. However, the nutritional advice given in the diet should enable the dieter to recognise restaurant dishes that will be high in complex carbohydrates and low in fat.

Exercise
The diet incorporates a comprehensive exercise plan to work in conjunction with the eating programme, and it is regarded as an integral part of successful fat burning.

Extras
The Fat Burning Diet also looks at some of the psychological aspects that motivate dieting and suggests that specific goals are determined. It also prepares the dieter for coping with the days when willpower is a little low and gives advice on controlling dietary addiction. The diet can be used in a moderated form, even after goal weight is achieved, as a permanent plan for healthy eating.

Full information about this diet is published in *The New Fat Burner Diet Book* by Patrick Holford and Bridget Woods (ION Press, 1995) £5.95. Also available is the *30-Day Fat Burner Diet* by Patrick Holford (Piatkus Books, 1999).

The New Biogenic Diet

THE New Biogenic Diet eschews the traditional calorie-counting approach to weight loss in favour of a new method of categorising foods through their ability to heal and revitalise the body. Based on an experiment that was begun in the 1920s, this diet operates on a more holistic basis whereby the promotion of detoxification in the body has various benefits for health, including the loss of excess weight.

Recommended for
Dieters who wish to combine gradual weight loss with the use of fresh and natural foods.

Not recommended for
The New Biogenic Diet is not ideal for anybody who wishes to achieve rapid weight loss on a more conventional calorie-controlled diet. The general philosophy behind the diet demands that fundamental and permanent changes are made to eating habits.

The process of removing toxic wastes from the fat cells of the body facilitates the restoration of the biochemical balance and the metabolic function to a high level of efficiency, thereby stimulating the burning of excess fat.

Traditionally we have been encouraged to analyse our diet in terms of the amount and balance of the five major nutrient groups – carbohydrates, proteins, fats, vitamins and minerals. The New Biogenic Diet, however, redefines these categorisations as follows:

- **Biogenic foods** – nuts, sprouted seeds, wholegrains and beans
- **Bioactive foods** – fresh fruits, vegetable, and herbs
- **Biostatic foods** – unprocessed cereal and wholegrain foods, free-range eggs and chicken, game meat and cooked vegetables and beans.
- **Biocidic foods** – highly processed, highly refined, high-fat foods.

The diet concentrates on combining foods in the **biogenic, bioactive** and **biostatic** groups; biocidic foods are not included as these will increase toxicity and interfere with a healthy metabolism. This means that approximately 75 per cent of the diet is derived from living foods (e.g. sprouting seeds), which promote the removal of waste products from the body and increase the efficiency of the metabolism.

However, it is the way in which these foods are combined which is important in this diet. Once food has been eaten, if it is not digested efficiently then the nutrients cannot be utilised properly, resulting in the build-up of toxins which are stored in the fat cells of the body. This can be caused by eating the wrong type of food or from combining foods which are dependent on different enzymes for their breakdown. For example, proteins need an acid medium for their breakdown, while starches (complex carbohydrates such as wholegrains, potatoes, cereals, and breads) require an alkaline medium. If these foods are eaten in combination then they cannot be broken down effectively and digestion will be incomplete, resulting in a production of toxins.

Most vegetables are neutral foods which can be broken down in either an alkaline or an acidic medium and can thus be combined with both starches and proteins. In this way the diet has certain principles and guidelines which, if followed, will promote this detoxification process.

- Do not mix concentrated proteins with concentrated starches in one meal. If you are planning to eat a protein meal and a starch meal on the same day then five hours should elapse between eating the meals.
- Eat only fruit for breakfast and always eat fruit on its own.
- Eat only one starch or one protein food per meal.
- Try to use foods which are as near as possible to their fresh, natural state.
- Do not eat biocidic foods (see above).

While this eating plan may initially appear complicated and restrictive, the New Biogenic Diet sets out a plan which simplifies the theory into practice with charts that clearly define the desirable food combinations along with specific lists of recommended foods. The eating plans for each day will enable the dieter to get used to this method of food combining, while taking advantage of appetising and imaginative recipes such as barley mushroom soup, grilled chicken breast with lemon parsnips, and mange tout and almond stir fry.

A typical day's menu
Breakfast
Fresh fruit or fruit salad

Lunch
Sprouted lentil salad *or* barley mushroom soup *or* spring greens salad

Dinner
Baked leeks and pecans with green glory salad *or* grilled chicken breast with lemon baked parsnips *or* easy vegetable curry with small sprout salad and Italian dressing

Eating out
The author makes general recommendations for eating out in restaurants and at dinner parties, while following this diet. This generally involves using your consumer power to ensure that the food you are served is biogenic. There are also tips for biogenic packed lunches.

There will be no calorific guideline for the dieter to stick to but the foods recommended by the diet are low fat and natural, with the advantage that they are filling and use moderate amounts of biostatic foods to create variety and interest.

How fast is it?
Weight loss is only one of the advantages of the New Biogenic Diet. It is fundamentally an approach to eating that will maximise bodily health and vitality. As such it has greater value if adopted as an eating philosophy as opposed to a limited regime for losing excess weight.

Exercise
Leslie Kenton recommends that exercise should be performed three to four times a week, and that it should be non-stop and sustained for a period of at least 40 minutes.

Full information about this diet is published in *The New Biogenic Diet* by Leslie Kenton (Vermillion, 1995) £8.99. Also available is the *Biogenic Food-Combining Diet* (Vermillion 2000).

Judith Wills' Complete Speed Slimming Plan

THIS is a weight loss programme that combines a calorie-controlled eating plan with an exercise plan to achieve rapid weight loss. The author of this diet believes that many diet programmes fail because the rate at which weight is lost is too gradual, leading the dieter to become demoralised and then throw in the towel.

Recommended for
Dieters who wish to lose weight rapidly.

Not recommended for
Anyone who is aged under 18 or over 65 years.

Speed slimming can be achieved and the weight-loss maintained without recourse to fad or crash-dieting. This involves the careful orchestration of a reduced-calorie eating plan with an exercise programme designed to boost the metabolism and concentrate on improving the shape of particular areas of the body.

Based around a nutritional balance of 65 to 70 per cent carbohydrate, 10 to 15 per cent protein and 20 per cent fat (of which only 10 per cent or less can be saturated fat) the diet plan works on a sliding-scale principle. There are five diet plans from which the dieter can choose, according to how much weight they wish to lose.

- Diet 1 – 42 lb (19 kg) or more to lose
- Diet 2 – 28 to 42 lb (12.7 to 19 kg) to lose
- Diet 3 – 14 to 28 lb (6.4 to 12.7 kg) to lose
- Diet 4 – 7 to 14 lb (3.2 to 6.4 kg) to lose
- Diet 5 – 7 lb (3.2 kg) or less to lose

In addition to this the dieter is required to answer a brief questionnaire that will define whether their metabolic rate is high, average or low. This is based on height, age, build, daily activity level, exercise level and personality.

The slimmer can use all this information to decide which of the five plans is the most appropriate. Once a dieter has lost a certain amount of weight he or she can then move on to the next diet; for example a dieter with 28 lb (12.7 kg) to lose will begin on Diet 3 and once he or she has lost 14 lb (6.4 kg) can then move on to Diet 4, to lose another 14 lb and so on, until target weight has been reached. There are two options within each diet plan:

- The **Set Diet** – recommended for dieters who feel that they need specific instruction and guidance
- The **Flexi Diet** – a multi-choice approach, recommended for dieters with specific needs, such as vegetarians.

Both diets can be used, so if the dieter feels more confident about managing her eating plan after a couple of weeks on the Set Diet she can then try the Flexi Diet in Week 3.

There is a list of unlimited vegetables that can be served at any time, and a fruit allowance for each day. In addition the dieter is allowed a 100-calorie snack allowance to be taken from a list of suggestions. Dieters with a high metabolism can take three snacks a day, those with an average metabolism are allowed two per day, and those with a low metabolism can choose one snack. It is recommended that at least one of these snacks is chosen from the fruit-based options.

Menu plans for each diet are given for a seven-day period and the portion sizes are specified – so you don't have to worry about counting calories for each meal suggestion.

A typical day's menu from Diet 3
Daily allowance
125 ml (4 fl oz) skimmed milk for use in tea and coffee, plus the specified snack allowance.
Breakfast
1 medium-sized boiled egg
1 slice of bread with a small amount of low-fat spread
Lunch
2 slices of bread with 100 g (3^1/$_2$ oz) cottage cheese, salad vegetables from the unlimited list and 1 tomato
1 small fruit

Evening meal

1 portion red pepper pasta with a green salad garnish

or

75 g (3 oz) tagliatelle (dry weight) with 1 portion of tomato sauce and 1 tablespoon of Parmesan cheese.

On the Flexi Diet the slimmer can choose from several options for each meal which ensures variety and the flexibility to pick meals that will fit in with personal needs, such as taking a packed lunch to work or preparing a meal that can be served to family or friends. There are a range of imaginative recipes that have been devised for the plan, including tuna and broccoli bake, vegetable rice, and nutty chicken with beansprouts.

Eating out

There is no specific advice on eating out. The diet does aim to re-educate eating habits in the long-term, with advice on food composition and methods of controlling eating behaviour.

How fast is it?

With the emphasis firmly on speed slimming, the author quotes the average weight loss as 5 to 7 lb (2.3 to 3.2 kg) in the first week and 3 to 4 lb (1.4 to 1.8 kg) per week thereafter. The total weight loss in the first week will include fluid as well as fat loss.

In addition, the Speed Plus Plan has been devised for dieters who have enjoyed a couple of days of indulgence and need a quick kick-start to get them back on course.

Based on a daily calorific intake of 800 calories (which is below the recommended minimum), the Speed Plus Plan is designed to be used as a very short term measure, in order to give the dieter a much needed psychological and physical boost. It should not be followed for more than five days.

Exercise

While the dieter will lose weight following the eating plan, exercise is integral to the whole speed approach of this diet. It will boost the metabolism and burn off fat more rapidly. There are two exercise programmes on this diet:

- The **Fat-burning** plan – sustained aerobic exercises for loss of fat
- The **Body-shaping** plan – exercises to shape, tone and strengthen muscles in particular areas of the body.

Before embarking on an exercise programme the dieter is taken through a series of questions and self-assessment instructions to help her choose which plan and level of exercise is most suitable.

The Fat-burning consists of a programme for walking and cycling exercises which gradually increase in speed and distance over a series of stages.

The Body-shaping plan has a core routine for warm-up, toning and cool-down exercises to which the dieter can add any of the supplementary exercises. These supplements concentrate on the following areas of the body: the chest, upper back and arms; the waist, stomach and lower back; the bottom, hips, thighs and calves. So, while improving general fitness and body tone you can also concentrate on improving the shape and tone in a specific area of the body.

Extras

Once target weight has been achieved, the dieter is encouraged to combine the eating habits established on the diet with the exercises to ensure that the new weight is maintained.

A transition programme has been devised to increase calorific intake over a 12-day period. This works by taking the dieter back through the sliding scale plans from Diet 5 to Diet 1.

Full information about this diet is published in *Judith Wills' Complete Speed Slimming Plan* by Judith Wills (Vermillion, 1993) £8.99. Also published is *High Speed Slimming* by Judith Wills (Vermillion, 1997).

The Carbohydrate Addict's Diet

T HE Carbohydrate Addict's Diet is a weight loss programme devised specifically for people who, it claims, suffer from a condition called 'hyperinsulaemia', whereby the consumption of carbohydrates causes an increase in appetite and cravings, which are at the heart of weight gain.

Recommended for
This diet is ideal for anybody who has experienced the frustration of 'yo-yo' dieting. If you have experienced any of the following symptoms it could be that you are a carbohydrate addict and need a weight loss plan specifically tailored to this problem.
- Feeling hungry or feeling the need to eat a couple of hours after a large meal
- Feeling very emotional, either euphoric or depressed, for no particular reason
- A feeling of fatigue or lassitude after eating
- A constant preoccupation with food and eating
- Feelings of anxiety, frustration and anger that, again, occur for no particular reason

Not recommended for
Carbohydrate addiction must not be confused with diabetes, which should be treated medically. If you do not experience any of the symptoms listed above then you should look at other weight loss programmes.

The condition of being overweight is related to a number of factors but insulin imbalance is frequently apparent. Carbohydrate addicts in particular suffer from a dysfunction in this area, which affects the core mechanism of appetite control.

Normally, when carbohydrates are consumed the body releases insulin in two phases. The first phase occurs within seconds of starting to eat, and the same amount is released every time. The second phase occurs after the substance is eaten and depends on how much carbohydrate is actually consumed. In a normal person the body releases just enough insulin to aid the delivery of the carbohydrate energy (glucose) to the liver, muscle tissue or fat cells. As the glucose is accepted the level of insulin in the blood drops and the brain chemical serotonin is released. It is this chemical which creates the feeling of satisfaction and dietary 'fullness' after a meal.

When insulin (known as the hunger hormone) is malfunctioning it can cause a disturbance to the eating pattern and create subsequent weight problems. The authors of this diet believe that the carbohydrate addict cannot control the amounts of insulin released, and when carbohydrates are eaten the body is flooded with an excess of the hormone. This overdose of insulin effects the normal absorption of glucose and inhibits the rise of serotonin in the brain. The addict is therefore unable to feel satisfied by the food intake, and continues to feel hungry. If carbohydrates are constantly consumed in an attempt to achieve satisfaction, there will be a perpetual increase in insulin levels and the craving for food.

Carbohydrate addicts are more likely to store fat and thus have a greater tendency to obesity, making appetite control vital in the fight for weight loss.

The diet provides questionnaires to allow the individual to assess his or her suitability for the diet and to improve their awareness of the reflex urge to eat. According to the authors of the diet there are progressive levels of addiction and different types of carbohydrates that aggravate the problem.

The main aim of the programme is to educate the dieter, who is often totally unaware of the addiction, and resolve the physical and psychological problems associated with carbohydrate addiction. This then establishes the basis for achieving permanent weight loss.

Addiction level 1

On this scale the addiction to carbohydrates is camouflaged by a general craving for all foods. Addicts often feel that they are following a healthy diet including wholegrains, lean meat, vegetables and potatoes, with which they are satisfied. They usually think they are in control and simply love food – but weight slowly rises.

Addiction level 2

At this level the focus narrows onto starches such as bread, pasta, rice and potatoes. They seem to become more important and satisfying, and snack food also gains prominence. However, the diet is still relatively healthy. Starchy food tends to produce a feeling of relaxation, but the effects are short lived and in time increasing amounts are needed to create the same response. At this point the addict starts to feel concerned about eating patterns and weight control.

Addiction level 3

Starchy foods maintain their importance, while sweet foods become increasingly attractive. Healthier foods are pushed out of the diet and most protein is only an accompaniment to carbohydrates. The dieter realises that the urge to eat occurs without feelings of hunger or even a desire to eat. It has become more of a compulsion and less of an enjoyment. The addict finds that traditional meal times disappear and food is eaten on frequent demand. The day becomes a continual snack. The addict complains of feeling helpless and completely unable to harness the inner demand to eat.

The addict progresses from level to level through emotional, hormonal and environmental triggers. Stress has a huge part to play in the escalation of the addiction.

The diet itself works on the premise that by reducing the intake of carbohydrates in the daily diet, it is easier to regulate the insulin-serotonin cycle. Addicts find it very difficult to control appetite when constantly eating carbohydrates and so, by reducing intake to say once a day, the cravings and urges subside and weight loss can be achieved.

There is no calorie counting or measuring; portions are used instead but are not limited in size. The dieter is not expected to give up favourite foods, as the idea of deprivation does not aid successful slimming. In the goal for permanent weight loss the diet helps the dieter work around the chemical idiosyncrasies in a way that would not be suitable for non-addicts, who can follow a more conventional calorie-controlled diet.

The eating programme is organised into a 14-day plan, each day of which includes two complementary and one reward meal. The order in which meals are taken during the day can be varied. The complementary meals are low-carbohydrate meals, and should consist of 4 to 6 oz (115 to 150 g) of meat or fish, 2 to 3 oz (60 to 90 g) of cheese, and 2 cups of vegetables or salad. These will satisfy the appetite and control insulin levels. Reward meals allow the dieter to eat a healthy balanced meal which includes carbohydrate. This helps in the control of excess insulin production and acts as an incentive for the dieter. The reward meal should be eaten within a period of one hour and any alcoholic drinks must be consumed during this meal.

The meal plans feature suggestions and recipes which will enable the dieter to get used to the balance of low-carbohydrate meals. In addition a list of recommended foods is provided for the complementary meals, along with guidelines for portion sizes.

A typical menu
Breakfast
Light and airy muffins
Lunch
Baked herb-marinated chicken served with a tossed green salad
Lemon heaven and iced tea
Dinner
A carbohydrate rich 'reward' meal, as desired

Eating out
General hints are given for eating out. It is suggested that a restaurant is the ideal environment for a carbohydrate-rich reward meal. Otherwise general hints are given on the types of menu choices that will be low in carbohydrate.

How fast is it?
The Carbohydrate Addict's Diet aims for a slow, steady, gradual weight loss – no expected rate of weight loss is cited by the authors.

Exercise
There is no exercise programme for the Carbohydrate Addict's Diet. However, the authors do recommend that you take part in a form of physical activity that you will find enjoyable—for successful weight loss and for general health.

Extras
General guidance is given for adjusting the diet for permanent control of carbohydrate addiction, once target weight has been reached. In addition

the authors use case histories to analyse the best strategies and techniques for succeeding with the weight-loss plan.

Full information about this diet is published in *The Carbohydrate Addict's Diet* by Dr Rachael F. Heller & Dr Richard F. Heller (Cedar, 1996) £6.99. Also available are *The Carbohydrate Addict's Healthy for Life* (Plume Books, 1996), *The Carbohydrate Addict's Program for Success* (Plume Books, 1993) both also by Dr Rachael F. Heller & Dr Richard F. Heller.

The Scarsdale Medical Diet

THE Scarsdale Medical Diet is based on a low-calorie eating programme, with most of the calories derived from protein. The diet is divided into two parts, an extremely low-calorie, rapid weight-loss plan which is followed for no more than two weeks, alternating with a somewhat higher calorie, more carbohydrate, slower weight loss, 'keep trim' programme.

Not recommended for
Not recommended for long term usage, as it does not promote a balanced diet.

The higher-calorie maintenance plan should be followed for at least two weeks before resuming the rapid weight-loss regime, if required. The low-calorie menus are fairly rigid although they can be swapped about as long as the basic plan is still followed. Fat and sugar-free sauces are permitted as are very low-calorie diet drinks, although alcohol is not permitted. No butter, margarine, cooking oils, mayonnaise, milk or sugar is permitted on the low-calorie programme. Recommended foods include lean meat with all fat removed, skinned poultry, green salad and some vegetables and raw carrot and celery, which can be eaten as often as desired.

A typical day's menu
Breakfast
Black coffee or tea with artificial sweetener, if required
Grapefruit
Lunch
Tuna and green salad
Portion of melon or grapefruit
Dinner
2 very lean pork chops, grilled
Mixed green salad
Black coffee or tea

The menus in the maintenance or 'keep trim' programme allow for greater variety and an increased allowance of calories in the form of carbohydrate and fibre. There is an adventurous, 'international' section giving details of recipes from around the world which are adapted to fit the Scarsdale diet plan. Although vegetarians and vegans are provided for in the programme, the reliance on fish and meat makes the Scarsdale plan more suitable for those who normally eat animal protein.

The dangers of high protein, low carbohydrate diets are detailed in the next chapter. They have been widely condemned by doctors and nutritionists as being nutritionally unsound.

Not Recommended

High-protein, low- or no-carbohydrate 'fad' diets

High protein diets first appeared in the 1970s and were soon being criticised by health and medical experts for being nutritionally unsound. These diets have recently resurfaced, some of them claiming to be new and others in a reworked form and have 'taken off' as the latest slimming craze. They are being followed by many thousands of people, especially in America, and some of these are celebrities whose actions tend to be copied by others. However, high-protein, no- or very low-carbohydrate diets continue to be almost universally condemned by doctors and nutritionists because they are dangerous to health. The detailed, scientific and medical arguments are complex but some of the criticisms of the diets and those who propose them are listed below:

1   Most of the people who promote the diets do not have a medical or scientific background or any training in, or understanding of, the complexities of human nutrition. They make spurious, 'pseudo-scientific' statements regarding digestion, enzymes, metabolism, the role of insulin and carbohydrates, etc, which sound convincing but are completely wrong. They frequently quote results of 'research' to support their statements when, in fact, the studies have either not been carried out or, if they have, refute their claims.

2   By excluding carbohydrates, high protein diets are inevitably unbalanced with a serious lack of vitamins, minerals, antioxidants and fibre. In some of the plans, supplements are recommended, sometimes marketed by those promoting the diet.

3   High protein, no carbohydrate diets are low in calories, just like other weight-loss plans, although they are not promoted as such. It is suggested that the dieter can eat all he or she wants of high protein foods whereas, in fact, amounts are controlled.

4   The diets encourage an almost exclusive consumption of protein foods of animal origin which inevitably contain a high proportion of fat,

especially saturated fat and cholesterol. These elements increase the long-term risk of heart and circulatory disease and, possibly, some forms of cancer.

5   The lack of fibre resulting from the exclusion of carbohydrates causes an increased likelihood of constipation and other digestive disorders such as Irritable Bowel Syndrome. A lack of dietary fibre is linked with the development of bowel cancer.

6   A high protein, no carbohydrate diet has a diuretic effect, causing the loss of water from the tissues, which may be greater than the normal loss that occurs with dieting. This may lead people to falsely believe that they are losing more body fat than is actually the case.

7   Ketogenesis is the normal production of organic compounds called ketones in the body, which occurs when fats are metabolised. If carbohydrates are lacking, the body turns to fat as an energy source and there is a greater than normal production of ketones. This eventually induces an abnormal state called ketosis, in which ketones appear in the blood and urine (ketonuria). Ketosis is interpreted by the body as a state of starvation and, as an emergency response, it may begin to break down protein in muscle tissue. Other symptoms include headaches, dehydration, faintness, irritability, sickness, kidney disorders and bad breath. As well as occurring as a result of fasting or starvation, ketosis is most frequently seen in diabetes mellitus when it can result in coma and death.

      Those who promote high protein/no carbohydrate diets advocate using the dangerous state of ketosis to lose weight. The dieter may need to use a colour indicator stick to check a urine sample each day to ensure that he or she is still in ketosis and thus utilising fat as an energy source. However, unseen damage may also be occurring at the same time, especially in susceptible individuals and all adherents to this dietary regime must put up with constant bad breath.

8   Undiagnosed diabetes mellitus is known to be prevalent in the British Isles and ketosis in these individuals could cause serious illness or death. In addition, ketosis in pregnancy can result in death or abnormality of the developing foetus, which may occur at an early stage.

9   High protein fad diets usually take no account of the importance of exercise in promoting weight loss and do not suggest a plan for returning to a normal, healthy pattern of eating. They have become very popular

and are being hailed by some people as a sort of 'wonder cure' for obesity. In North America, where the diets have attracted a huge following, it is estimated that half the population is obese. This is mainly because Americans eat enormous quantities of high fat foods and have, on average, an even more sedentary lifestyle than people in Western Europe. In restaurants and cafés, portion sizes tend to be huge and served on large plates to accommodate the amount of food. Research has shown that most Americans have no idea what a portion size should be or how much they should be eating and greatly underestimate their actual calorie intake. The manner in which high protein fad diets are promoted does nothing to educate people about why they are obese or to encourage them to take personal responsibility by exercising self-control.

10 Most experts in nutrition believe that a largely plant-based diet, with occasional consumption of animal protein and foods eaten in as natural a state as possible, is the one which has the greatest benefits for health. This is the type of diet that is followed by many people in non-western countries where there are low rates of obesity and heart disease. It is evident that high protein, no or low carbohydrate diets are about as far removed from this as they can possibly be. Hence, although they do seem to result in weight loss, they cannot be recommended because of their adverse, long-term effects upon health.

Meal replacement diets

There are very many meal replacement products on the market, designed as slimming aids and generally for short-term use only. The products take the form of drinks or soups – usually freeze-dried, to be reconstituted in hot or cold water – or bars, all in a variety of flavours, calorie-reduced and nutritionally balanced, generally containing recommended amounts of vitamins and minerals. Meal replacement products are usually widely available from chemists and pharmacies but tend to be fairly expensive and overall costs may be quite high. Quite often meal replacement plans are in two stages with, perhaps, one week of strict adherence to meal replacements followed by a regime of limited use of the products and eating normal, low-calorie meals. Lists of permitted and banned foods are usually supplied, along with general dietary advice.

In this way, a programme of fairly rapid weight loss is achieved with, generally, an advice sheet on healthy eating once the target weight has been reached. These plans all advocate drinking plenty of water – at least six to eight glasses a day – to avoid the risk of dehydration and contain fairly detailed dietary advice. Some may advise a medical check-up before embarking upon the plan and also contain information on people who should not use the products.

Meal replacement diets often find favour with people seeking a short-term weight loss over a limited period who do not want to bother with calorie counting, weighing out portions or specialised cookery. While many people feel it is easy to follow the plan and enjoy the flavours that are on offer, others find them unappetising and boring. Meal replacement diets become difficult to follow when this is the case and in this instance it is probably better to choose a more varied type of slimming diet.

Slimming pills and dietary aids

The multi-million pound slimming industry truly comes into its own in the production, promotion and marketing of innumerable types of pills, patches and sprays, all claiming (unless you read the small print), to make people thin! Most of these products are not recommended by health professionals and many lack the scientific data to support their claims. Some of the pills contain powerful drugs which may or may not act as appetite suppressants but which can, in any event, have potentially harmful side effects. The most useful advice is not to believe all the exaggerated claims that are made by the manufacturers of slimming preparations, but if you wish to use them consult your doctor on the advisability of doing so. It is certainly the case that diet pills tend to be expensive and there are likely to be simpler and more enjoyable ways to slim.

Single food diets

Single food diets, usually based on eating, for example, one particular type of fruit for a set period of time, are basically the same as undertaking fasting as a means of weight loss. They are evidently nutritionally unsound and can be dangerous, producing vitamin and mineral deficiencies and damage to body organs, including the heart, which may be irreversible. In the short term, the unpleasant symptoms produced by such a regime are the same as those of fasting, e.g. headache, light-headedness, nausea, dizziness, feeling cold, tiredness, constipation, dry skin and dull hair.

Fasting

Fasting, in its strictest sense, means going without food altogether and only drinking liquids. It is a practice which has been known to many human societies for thousands of years and was usually undertaken for spiritual and religious reasons. However, fasting in this context was usually strictly controlled, limited in time and did not necessarily involve complete abstinence from food. Also, it was not always undertaken by every member of the community but often only by spiritual leaders. As with single food diets, and for all the same reasons, fasting as a means of achieving weight loss is a dangerous practice.

It is sometimes prescribed, under strict medical supervision, for very obese people who have perhaps tried and failed to lose weight by more conventional means and whose health is judged to be at risk. However, fasting in this context, which usually takes place within hospital, does not mean withdrawal of all nutrition. Instead, the patient is placed on a liquid protein diet and supplied with vitamin and mineral supplements, with constant monitoring both of overall health and weight loss to ensure that all is well. Fasting to bring about weight loss should never be attempted alone.

Summary and Conclusions

T HIS book is intended to provide a broad overview of one particular aspect, of human health – the importance of maintaining a reasonable body weight. It highlights the fact that it is impossible to discuss body weight in isolation as it is so intricately connected with many other aspects of physical and psychological health. It has been shown that this is particularly the case in Western countries where, in spite of the fact that people are becoming ever larger, a cultural ideal of extreme thinness is promoted.

The powerful and destructive influence of the cultural stereotype is discussed in relation to a rising rate in the incidence of eating disorders. The fact that excessive thinness is both unhealthy and unobtainable for normal people is also discussed. Acceptance of the concept of female beauty equating with thinness is a recent phenomenon. From historical times until comparatively recently, a plumper, rounder ideal of female beauty was applauded. This may have been partly due to the fact that it was considered important for women to produce children. It was probably recognized that a thin, underweight female was much more likely to suffer problems of infertility – and this remains the case today.

Paradoxically, set against the cultural promotion of thinness, all Western countries are experiencing an escalation in the number of their population who are either overweight or obese. This book examines in some detail the role of food and nutrition and seeks to explain why more and more people are becoming fat. The importance of eating a healthy, balanced diet to promote good health is discussed and lifestyle factors are examined in relation to the problem of gaining weight. The health, social and psychological problems experienced by some overweight and obese people, which can be intensified by the pervading cultural climate, are explored. However, positive factors are also emphasized, particularly that some larger people who are happy with their size are now 'fighting back' and asserting their right to be as they are without interference or criticism from others.

The book examines the operation of two factors involved in eating, appetite and hunger which are found to be complex mechanisms that are imperfectly understood and may vary between different people. There is a great deal of psychological and cultural 'baggage' attached to food and the whole business of eating. This is analysed to see how it might affect a person's weight and, more particularly, the way these factors may affect someone who is attempting to diet. Eating disorders are described in detail as they are so closely linked with the culturally-driven pressure to be slim and hence with dieting. It is felt that everyone needs to be aware of the risks and dangers of eating disorders, particularly if they have any involvement with young people.

Genetic factors affecting body weight are the subject of considerable scientific research and these are discussed, along with some interesting new findings recently announced in the media. It is felt that while genetic factors are undoubtedly important, the diet and lifestyle of each individual is probably of greater significance in controlling his or her weight. A considerable portion of the book is devoted to helping the reader to discover whether he or she really is overweight and should therefore consider going on a diet. The most reliable tests for finding this out are presented in the text and readers who are slightly overweight may be pleasantly surprised to discover that there is no reason why they should diet on health grounds alone!

An understanding of how the body reacts to a restricted food intake is important for successful dieting and so this, along with the role of exercise, is presented in this book. Lack of physical activity is felt to be one of the main contributory factors in the rising incidence of obesity in Western countries. The point is made that there is a form of exercise suitable for everyone and that it is important for all people to be as physically active as possible, whether they need to lose weight or not. A personal self-assessment is helpful in sorting out likes and dislikes with regard to food and eating and in discovering one's attitude to losing weight. These factors are explored with a view to giving guidance on choosing a suitable diet plan which will result in the best chance of success. Finally, ways to succeed in dieting and for keeping the weight off once it has been lost are discussed before introducing and evaluating some of the diet plans that are currently available.

This book has tried to do more than merely list and describe diet plans. An attempt has been made to cover all the health issues, both physical and psychological, attached to obesity, dieting and weight loss. Above all, in an age when we are all bombarded with information from many different quarters, the book has tried to pin down exactly what constitutes healthy eating and a healthy lifestyle. In the modern age, perhaps more than at any time in the past, people seek to be well-informed about any disease, illness or medical condition that affects their health. However, weight control is perhaps the only aspect of health that has had a multi-million pound industry built up around it, where fortunes can and have been made by the introduction of a new fad diet or wonder, weight loss pill!

Of course, the counterside of this is the very many people who have lost money on failed diets and who remain disappointed and the same size and weight as they were before. Hence knowledge for the would-be dieter is extremely important and it is hoped that this book will help you to be 'forewarned and forearmed' and, above all, helped to succeed if you wish to lose weight. Good dieting!

III

Your Personal Healthy Eating and Exercise Plan

Your Six-Month
Personal Plan

A DIET journal is a good idea because if you write down your goal you are rather more inclined to follow it through. Before you begin to write your plan you should read the advice on nutrition, exercise, determining the need to diet, and our reviews of popular diets. If you haven't done that please go back and read those sections now, it is very important that you do so.

A combination of balanced diet, aerobic exercise and positive mental attitude are all you need, in theory, to lose weight and be healthy.

This plan is for six months. It contains charts, graphs and a journal to take note of your progress. If at any point you feel you are not progressing as positively as you had hoped then this plan should enable you to go back over your journal and pinpoint where you are going wrong, or whether there has been anything happening in your life that is hindering your progress.

If you feel that calorie counting is boring and not for you then that's fine, but remember to stick to your healthy balance of eating complex carbohydrate for energy, protein for lean muscle, a little fat and lots of fruit, vegetables and fibre for vitamins, vitality and digestive health. After six months you should know your healthy eating and exercise routine inside out and be able to carry it out without writing it down.

Calorie intake and metabolism

Remember that those of you who are considerably overweight will be able to lose weight consuming more calories than those of you who are just a little overweight. Contrary to the popular belief that people are fat because of a slow metabolism, actually, fat people have faster metabolisms than those who are naturally slim.

Overweight people, in general, also have more quantities of muscle tissue than slim people. This is because it takes effort and more energy to move around with that extra weight. An overweight person will burn more calories than a slim person during identical exercise regimes (see the table on pages 75–96 for how many calories are burned during different activities for people of different weights. On page 66 we showed you how to work out your basal metabolic rate. As you lose weight, keep a record of this and your body mass index (charts on pages 55–60).

As you lose weight your metabolism may slow down. To contend with this you must ensure that you eat sensibly and exercise so that you do not lose too much lean muscle tissue. Lean muscle tissue is fat-burning tissue. As you lose weight you will feel more energetic and this will help you to progress in your exercise plan. It is normal to gain a little weight after you reach your goal weight and start to eat normally again. Don't be discouraged, just keep putting your new eating habits into practice.

How quickly should you lose weight?
Most health professionals recommend that you lose 1 to 2 lbs per week. If you combine this with an exercise plan and the use of light weights, this may help to keep the muscles toned and avoid the saggy skin that can sometimes follow weight loss. See pages 69 to 76 for advice on the recommended amount of exercise that you should follow.

Judith Wills, in her book *High Speed Slimming*, insists that there is no hard evidence to show that losing weight quickly is harmful. She argues that it is more encouraging to see quick results, especially in those who are very overweight, than to struggle away for months with little progress. Her book recommends that you exercise a lot to increase the metabolism, eat a healthy, balanced diet in sufficient amounts to maintain your lean muscle tissue and become informed about what you eat. You must never starve yourself. Ask your doctor for his or her advice about such following such a plan. Remember, too much exercise can also be harmful.

Losing weight quickly without re-educating yourself about your diet and without taking care to ask yourself why you eat too much will be disastrous. That is why meal-substitute plans, fad diets and weird food combinations are rarely long-term solutions because it's all too easy to go back to your old habits when you finally crack and can't bear the deprivation any longer.

I'm bored with my plan!
If you are bored with a health plan then it may be the wrong one for you.

Why are you bored? Are you eating the same things all the time? Are you following the same exercise plan week after week? Are you exercising on your own? Are you losing weight too slowly?

Write down your favourite healthy foods. Learn new recipes that use them. You don't have to eat broccoli and spinach if you don't like them, but find something equally nutritious that you do enjoy. Do you hate boiled veggies? Spray them with very little garlic-infused olive oil and baste with basamic vinegar and a little honey, sprinkle them with some fresh herbs and sea salt and roast in the oven or barbecue them. Delicious!

If you hate the gym, and a lot of exercise environments are hardly inspiring, why not take a dance class or join a walking group? If your exercise time is more sociable it will be twice as enjoyable.

Do not starve yourself – it doesn't work

- Eating too little on a diet will create a vicious circle of weight loss and gain.
- Eating too little will make you cranky.
- Eating too little will do you physical harm; you will lose lean muscle tissue and your metabolism will slow down. Your blood sugar will drop and your body will go into starvation mode; it will release levels of potentially damaging adrenaline.
- Eat too little and you are denying yourself the vitamins and essential minerals that keep your skin, hair, and nails looking healthy and attractive.

If you deny yourself food to the point of starvation you are more likely to binge-eat and feel terrible about yourself afterwards, than if you carefully prepare for yourself a delicious, healthy, balanced meal that actually gives you energy and vitality.

Get interested in food and cooking

Food is fuel and food is fun.

Low calorie ready-made meals are convenient but hardly inspiring. They are often low in vitamins and fibre and high in highly-processed carbohydrates that are converted into glucose very quickly. Eating convenience food like this means that your blood sugar takes a plunge very quickly after you've eaten it, you produce adrenaline, and you want to eat more almost immediately.

Here's a little experiment (not recommended for diabetics). For breakfast one morning eat something high in quickly-absorbed carbohydrate (like a

Danish pastry, a croissant, or even rice cakes, because although rice cakes are very low-calorie, they have quite a high glycemic index (see page 119). Rice cakes have a GI of 82 – that's higher than that of sucrose which is 65! The croissant has a GI of 67. After eating any of these for breakfast, by mid-morning you will be ravenous! Shortly after eating food like this your blood sugar will rise very rapidly and then plummet. If you have porridge, Special K or All Bran and fruit, or some wholegrain rye bread and a scrape of butter instead, then that should keep you going till it's time for lunch because the carbohydrate in these foods is slowly absorbed and this keeps your bood sugar levels stable.

In other words, it's not the number of calories you consume that dictates how full up or hungry you will be, it's the kind of calories. (See *The Glucose Revolution*, Jennie Brand-Miller et al, for the best explanation of this and an excellent comprehensive listing of the glycemic index of foods).

Low-calorie convenience foods and substitutes also often don't taste that great. Also, some products imply that they are diet products but are far from it. Food labelled '80% fat free' may sound healthy, but what if they had labelled the product with 'contains 20% fat'? That doesn't sound quite so virtuous. Things that have a diet label on them are not necessarily good for you. If they are low in sugar they may be high in fat or sweeteners. If they are low in fat they may be high in sugar or salt or monosodium glutamate.

It is far, far better to take a real interest in your nutrition and to try to cook interesting, healthy food.

In your plan there is space to record some healthy recipes. Build up your repertoire of low-fat and nutritious meals. There is not space here to include a healthy-eating cookery course but there are plenty of excellent cookery books on the market that will point you in the right direction. There are also lots of sources of low fat recipes on the internet.

Fats and oils

Many diet plans are low in fat. Everyone agrees that too much fat in the diet is not good for you. Research has also shown, however, that no-fat diets are also bad for you, and some dietitians believe that small amounts of fat at certain times actually help curb your appetite.

So don't cut out that teaspoonful of olive oil or mayonnaise on your salad if you feel it makes it so much more palatable. If you want some chocolate, don't torture yourself, you'll just become obsessed by the thought of it. Have a little chocolate and compensate by being a little more active that day.

Some foods that are traditionally avoided by dieters are extremely good for us. Nuts are high in fat but are good for us because they are rich in vitamins, minerals and unsaturated fatty acids, so can help to lower cholesterol. Avocado is quite high in fat but is also good for the heart because it contains unsaturated fatty acids, which lower cholesterol, vitamin D and potassium, and has such a low glycemic index that you can count it as zero. It would seem sensible then to eat them in moderation but not to exclude them entirely from our diets.

Don't get obsessed

Try not to get obsessed by calorie counting. Organisations such as Weight Watchers are great if calorie counting bores you and eventually makes you go off your diet. They give you realistic meal and snack ideas. They also give you a bit of moral support to keep you on course and you'll meet people in the same boat as yourself.

Concentrate on good nutrition and good food theory (like the glycemic index) and balance your physical activity with the amounts and types of food you eat, so that no food is ever completely banned.

Calorie counting is not a waste of time but there are other ways of scrutinising the food we eat, so do take an interest in nutrition and follow the advice in the introductory chapters of this book.

If you do some calorie counting initially you will eventually be able to judge calorie content approximately just from the weight and ingredients of food, and this is probably accurate enough for our purposes. Don't cheat though!

Is fat the only issue?

Do you really need to diet? If you are fit and healthy, and people are always telling you that you don't need to lose weight, could it be that you just need to feel more positive about yourself?

Conversely, if someone is telling you that they think you are too fat, have you thought about your own feelings on the subject? Is this person a positive influence in your life or are they criticising you because of their own inadequacies or out of a need to bring you down to their level?

Do you overeat because you are bored? Maybe you need to find some more interests. Join a group, do a course, plan nights out with friends and try to do something new each time. It could ignite an interest that changes your life.

Do you often think: 'If only I was thinner I would have succeeded'? Some people use being overweight as an excuse when they fail, whether that is in a relationship or a friendship or in their career. Is being fat really the problem? Be honest, are there other aspects of your life where there are problems but you are too scared, or just not yet able, to deal with them? It is very important that you address these problems whether it be through a counsellor, your doctor or through talking to a close friend.

Do you overeat because you are unhappy? Do you avoid food to punish yourself? If so, then following a diet is never the answer. It is vital that you address your unhappiness by going to a counsellor or by talking to someone close about it. No diet is ever going to solve a problem like this – don't believe in any plan that promises miracles.

- Losing weight should be about improving your life and your health.
- Losing weight is not about trying to look like someone else.
- Losing weight is not about trying to please someone else.
- Losing weight will not necessarily make you more popular.
- Losing weight will not necessarily make you irresistible to the opposite sex.
- Losing weight will not make you more interesting (especially not if you bore your friends with the calorie content of all the foods they eat!)
- Losing weight will not necessarily make you happier.

For the very overweight, losing a lot of weight is sometimes just the first step on their road to good health. Sometimes if one person in a couple accomplishes a huge weight loss the other finds it difficult to adjust to and cope with their partner's new look and new confidence. It can threaten their own role and their security within that relationship.

Remember

Eating wonderful food is one of life's seriously great pleasures – but that's the key here, that it is just one of them! Food should only inhabit a small section of your life, you don't have to think about it all the time. Your family, partner, friends and social life, the friends you are yet to make, work, exercise, hobbies, interests – you need to make room for them all and not place undue importance on your own body image or use food as a crutch when something goes wrong in one of those areas.

Have fun making your plan as interesting as possible and remember to fit in lots of time for your friends, family and for your interests.

Graph of body mass index (BMI) over six months

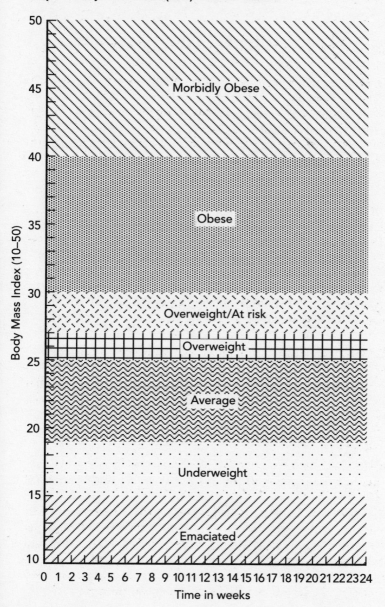

My Goals for Month One

During the first month of my healthy eating plan:

I want to reach my target weight of __45kg.__ (remember 1–2 lbs per week is recommended by most dieticians).

My body mass index is __22__.

My basal metabolic rate is __1210__ kilocalories per day.

I will take up a form of exercise that holds my interest and do it for a sustained period, at least twice a week.
Kinds of exercise I could investigate:

__Horseriding.__
__Running__
__Rollerblading.__

❏ I will also use light weights to build up my lean muscle tissue (It is best to do this with supervision at your local gym).

❏ I will spend more time with my friends and less time in front of the TV.

❏ I will spend around 30 minutes a day doing a mildly aerobic activity.

❏ I will learn more about the food I am eating.

❏ I will learn to cook, from scratch, 2 healthy meals which are fabulously tasty and low in fat, and write the recipes in my journal.

❑ I will talk about my problems and not bottle them up.

❑ If I can afford it I will try to fit in a reward, such as an aromatherapy massage, for following my plan. (Massage has been shown to be an aid to weight loss as well as an aid to stress.)

I will focus on my strengths which are:

_____
_____
_____
_____
_____
_____
_____
_____

I will identify the stresses in my life and try to avoid them or to find a way to relax to alleviate the stress.

_____
_____
_____
_____
_____
_____
_____

What triggers my overeating?
Here is a list of situations where I wasn't hungry yet found myself eating:

Boredom.
Eating when my boyfriend eats.
_____
_____
_____
_____

Week 1

From .... to ....

BMR .... Weight .... Goal ....

		Calories
Day 1		
	Activity	
Day 2		Calories
	Activity	
Day 3		Calories
	Activity	
Day 4		Calories
	Activity	
Day 5		Calories
	Activity	
Day 6		Calories
	Activity	
Day 7		Calories
	Activity	

Week 2

From .... to ....

BMR .... Weight .... Goal ....

		Calories
Day 8	Activity	
Day 9	Activity	Calories
Day 10	Activity	Calories
Day 11	Activity	Calories
Day 12	Activity	Calories
Day 13	Activity	Calories
Day 14	Activity	Calories

Week 3

From .... to ....

BMR .... Weight .... Goal ....

Day 15		Calories
	Activity	

Day 16		Calories
	Activity	

Day 17		Calories
	Activity	

Day 18		Calories
	Activity	

Day 19		Calories
	Activity	

Day 20		Calories
	Activity	

Day 21		Calories
	Activity	

Week 4

From .... to ....

BMR .... Weight .... Goal ....

Day 22		Calories
	Activity	
Day 23		Calories
	Activity	
Day 24		Calories
	Activity	
Day 25		Calories
	Activity	
Day 26		Calories
	Activity	
Day 27		Calories
	Activity	
Day 28		Calories
	Activity	

My Recipes

My Recipes

Shopping List

○

○

○

○

○

Activities

○

○

○

○

○

Negative Thoughts

○

○

○

○

○

Positive Thoughts

Calorie Record

My BMR is .... kilocalories per day

Day	Date	Morning	Afternoon	Evening	Total
Monday					
Tuesday					
Wednesday					
Thursday					
Friday					
Saturday					
Sunday					

Calorie Record

My BMR is .... kilocalories per day

Day	Date	Morning	Afternoon	Evening	Total
Monday					
Tuesday					
Wednesday					
Thursday					
Friday					
Saturday					
Sunday					

Your Personal Healthy Eating and Exercise Plan

Calorie Record

Day	Date	Morning	Afternoon	Evening	Total
Monday					
Tuesday					
Wednesday					
Thursday					
Friday					
Saturday					
Sunday					

My BMR is .... kilocalories per day

Calorie Record

My BMR is .... kilocalories per day

Day	Date	Morning	Afternoon	Evening	Total
Monday					
Tuesday					
Wednesday					
Thursday					
Friday					
Saturday					
Sunday					

My Goals for Month Two

During the second month of my healthy eating plan:

I want to reach my target weight of_____ .

My body mass index is _____ .

My basal metabolic rate is _____ kilocalories per day.

❑   I reached my target weight last month.

❑   I will continue to exercise at least twice a week.

❑   I will also use light weights to build up my lean muscle tissue.

❑   I will investigate other forms of activity such as a dance class, a walking group or a yoga class, in which I can participate with friends and also meet new people.

❑   I will learn to cook another 2 tasty low-fat meals and enter them in my journal.

❑   I will spend around 30 minutes a day doing a mildly aerobic activity.

❑   If I can afford it I will try to fit in a suitable reward for following my plan.

The problems I experienced last month that hindered my diet plan were:

_____
_____
_____
_____
_____
_____
_____
_____

How I can avoid or deal with these problems:

_____
_____
_____
_____
_____
_____
_____

What triggers my overeating?
Here is a list of situations where I wasn't hungry yet found myself eating:

_____
_____
_____
_____
_____
_____
_____

Week 5

From .... to ....

BMR .... Weight .... Goal ....

		Calories
Day 29	Activity	Calories
Day 30	Activity	Calories
Day 31	Activity	Calories
Day 32	Activity	Calories
Day 33	Activity	Calories
Day 34	Activity	Calories
Day 35	Activity	Calories

Week 6

From .... to ....

BMR .... Weight .... Goal ....

Day 36		Calories
	Activity	

Day 37		Calories
	Activity	

Day 38		Calories
	Activity	

Day 39		Calories
	Activity	

Day 40		Calories
	Activity	

Day 41		Calories
	Activity	

Day 42		Calories
	Activity	

Week 7

From .... to ....

BMR .... Weight .... Goal ....

Day 43		Calories
	Activity	

Day 44		Calories
	Activity	

Day 45		Calories
	Activity	

Day 46		Calories
	Activity	

Day 47		Calories
	Activity	

Day 48		Calories
	Activity	

Day 49		Calories
	Activity	

Week 8

From ....   to ....

BMR .... Weight .... Goal ....

Day 50		Calories
	Activity	

Day 51		Calories
	Activity	

Day 52		Calories
	Activity	

Day 53		Calories
	Activity	

Day 54		Calories
	Activity	

Day 55		Calories
	Activity	

Day 56		Calories
	Activity	

My Recipes

My Recipes

○

○

○

○

○

Shopping List

Activities

○

○

○

○

○

Negative Thoughts

Positive Thoughts

○

○

○

○

○

Your Personal Healthy Eating and Exercise Plan

Calorie Record

Day	Date	Morning	Afternoon	Evening	Total
Monday					
Tuesday					
Wednesday					
Thursday					
Friday					
Saturday					
Sunday					

My BMR is .... kilocalories per day

Calorie Record

My BMR is .... kilocalories per day

Day	Date	Morning	Afternoon	Evening	Total
Monday					
Tuesday					
Wednesday					
Thursday					
Friday					
Saturday					
Sunday					

Your Personal Healthy Eating and Exercise Plan

Calorie Record

My BMR is .... kilocalories per day

Day	Date	Morning	Afternoon	Evening	Total
Monday					
Tuesday					
Wednesday					
Thursday					
Friday					
Saturday					
Sunday					

Calorie Record

My BMR is .... kilocalories per day

Day	Date	Morning	Afternoon	Evening	Total
Monday					
Tuesday					
Wednesday					
Thursday					
Friday					
Saturday					
Sunday					

My Goals for Month Three

During the third month of my healthy eating plan:

I want to reach my target weight of _____ .

My body mass index is _____ .

My basal metabolic rate is _____ kilocalories per day.

❑   I reached my target weight last month.

I will continue to exercise at least twice a week, but I am now going to change my exercise plan as follows to keep it fresh:

_____

_____

_____

_____

_____

_____

❑   I will slightly increase the weights that I use to build up my lean muscle tissue.

❑   If I can afford it I will buy myself a new outfit as a reward for my weight loss (maybe a stylish new one for the gym to aid my confidence).

❑   I will make an effort to speak to a new person every time I go to the gym/exercise class/slimming class.

❑   I will learn to cook another 2 tasty low-fat meals and enter them in my journal.

❏ I will spend around 30 minutes a day doing a mildly aerobic activity.

❏ If I can afford it, I will try to fit in a suitable reward for following my plan.

The problems I experienced last month that hindered my diet plan were:

_____
_____
_____
_____
_____
_____
_____
_____

How I can avoid or deal with these problems:

_____
_____
_____
_____
_____
_____
_____

What triggers my overeating?
Here is a list of situations where I wasn't hungry yet found myself eating:

_____
_____
_____
_____
_____
_____
_____

Week 9

From ....   to ....

BMR .... Weight .... Goal ....

Day 57		Calories
	Activity	

Day 58		Calories
	Activity	

Day 59		Calories
	Activity	

Day 60		Calories
	Activity	

Day 61		Calories
	Activity	

Day 62		Calories
	Activity	

Day 63		Calories
	Activity	

Week 10

From .... to ....

BMR .... Weight .... Goal ....

		Calories
Day 64		
	Activity	
Day 65		Calories
	Activity	
Day 66		Calories
	Activity	
Day 67		Calories
	Activity	
Day 68		Calories
	Activity	
Day 69		Calories
	Activity	
Day 70		Calories
	Activity	

Week 11

From .... to ....

BMR .... Weight .... Goal ....

Day 71		Calories
	Activity	

Day 72		Calories
	Activity	

Day 73		Calories
	Activity	

Day 74		Calories
	Activity	

Day 75		Calories
	Activity	

Day 76		Calories
	Activity	

Day 77		Calories
	Activity	

Week 12

From .... to ....

BMR .... Weight .... Goal ....

Day 78		Calories
	Activity	

Day 89		Calories
	Activity	

Day 80		Calories
	Activity	

Day 81		Calories
	Activity	

Day 82		Calories
	Activity	

Day 83		Calories
	Activity	

Day 84		Calories
	Activity	

My Recipes

My Recipes

Shopping list

○

○

○

○

○

Activities

Negative Thoughts

Positive Thoughts

○

○

○

○

○

Your Personal Healthy Eating and Exercise Plan

Calorie Record

My BMR is .... kilocalories per day

Day	Date	Morning	Afternoon	Evening	Total
Monday					
Tuesday					
Wednesday					
Thursday					
Friday					
Saturday					
Sunday					

Calorie Record

My BMR is .... kilocalories per day

Day	Date	Morning	Afternoon	Evening	Total
Monday					
Tuesday					
Wednesday					
Thursday					
Friday					
Saturday					
Sunday					

Your Personal Healthy Eating and Exercise Plan

Calorie Record

My BMR is .... kilocalories per day

Day	Date	Morning	Afternoon	Evening	Total
Monday					
Tuesday					
Wednesday					
Thursday					
Friday					
Saturday					
Sunday					

Calorie Record

My BMR is .... kilocalories per day

Day	Date	Morning	Afternoon	Evening	Total
Monday					
Tuesday					
Wednesday					
Thursday					
Friday					
Saturday					
Sunday					

My Goals for Month Four

During the fourth month of my healthy eating plan:

I want to reach my target weight of _____ .

My body mass index is _____ .

My basal metabolic rate is _____ kilocalories per day

❑   I reached my target weight last month.

❑   I will continue to exercise at least twice a week.

❑   I will also use light weights to build up my lean muscle tissue.

❑   I will try to spend a complete hour, whenever I can, completely relaxing, without thinking about children, partner or work, focusing on the positive results of my healthy eating plan.

❑   I will learn to cook another 2 tasty low fat meals and enter them in my journal.

❑   I will spend around 30 minutes a day doing a mildly aerobic activity.

❑   If I can afford it I will try to fit in a suitable reward for following my plan.

The problems I experienced last month which hindered my diet plan were:

_____

_____

_____

_____

_____

_____

_____

_____

How I can avoid or deal with these problems:

_____

_____

_____

_____

_____

_____

_____

What triggers my overeating?
Here is a list of situations where I wasn't hungry yet found myself eating:

_____

_____

_____

_____

_____

_____

_____

Week 13

From .... to ....

BMR .... Weight .... Goal ....

Day 85		Calories
	Activity	

Day 86		Calories
	Activity	

Day 87		Calories
	Activity	

Day 88		Calories
	Activity	

Day 89		Calories
	Activity	

Day 90		Calories
	Activity	

Day 91		Calories
	Activity	

Week 14

From .... to ....

BMR .... Weight .... Goal ....

Day 92		Calories
	Activity	

Day 93		Calories
	Activity	

Day 94		Calories
	Activity	

Day 95		Calories
	Activity	

Day 96		Calories
	Activity	

Day 97		Calories
	Activity	

Day 98		Calories
	Activity	

Week 15

From ....   to ....

BMR .... Weight .... Goal ....

Day 99		Calories
	Activity	

Day 100		Calories
	Activity	

Day 101		Calories
	Activity	

Day 102		Calories
	Activity	

Day 103		Calories
	Activity	

Day 104		Calories
	Activity	

Day 105		Calories
	Activity	

Week 16

From ....   to ....

BMR ....   Weight ....   Goal ....

Day 106		Calories
	Activity	

Day 107		Calories
	Activity	

Day 108		Calories
	Activity	

Day 109		Calories
	Activity	

Day 110		Calories
	Activity	

Day 111		Calories
	Activity	

Day 112		Calories
	Activity	

My Recipes

My Recipes

Shopping List

Activities

○

○

○

○

○

Negative Thoughts

○

○

○

○

○

Positive Thoughts

○

○

○

○

○

Calorie Record

My BMR is .... kilocalories per day

Day	Date	Morning	Afternoon	Evening	Total
Monday					
Tuesday					
Wednesday					
Thursday					
Friday					
Saturday					
Sunday					

Calorie Record

My BMR is .... kilocalories per day

Day	Date	Morning	Afternoon	Evening	Total
Monday					
Tuesday					
Wednesday					
Thursday					
Friday					
Saturday					
Sunday					

Your Personal Healthy Eating and Exercise Plan

Calorie Record

My BMR is .... kilocalories per day

Day	Date	Morning	Afternoon	Evening	Total
Monday					
Tuesday					
Wednesday					
Thursday					
Friday					
Saturday					
Sunday					

Month Four

Calorie Record

My BMR is .... kilocalories per day

Day	Date	Morning	Afternoon	Evening	Total
Monday					
Tuesday					
Wednesday					
Thursday					
Friday					
Saturday					
Sunday					

My Goals for Month Five

During the fifth month of my healthy eating plan:

I want to reach my target weight of _____ .

My body mass index is _____ .

My basal metabolic rate is _____ kilocalories per day.

❏   I reached my target weight last month.

I will continue to exercise at least twice a week, but I am now going to change my exercise plan as follows to keep it fresh:

_____
_____
_____
_____
_____
_____
_____
_____

❏   I will slightly increase the weights that I use to build up my lean muscle tissue.

❏   I will learn to cook another 2 tasty low-fat meals.

❏   I will review all of the new recipes I have learned to cook and have friends over for a dinner party.

❏   I will spend around 30 minutes a day doing a mildly aerobic activity.

❏ If I can afford it I will try to fit in a suitable reward for following my plan.

The problems I experienced last month which hindered my diet plan were:

_____
_____
_____
_____
_____
_____
_____
_____

How I can avoid or deal with these problems:

_____
_____
_____
_____
_____
_____
_____
_____

What triggers my overeating?
Here is a list of situations where I wasn't hungry yet found myself eating:

_____
_____
_____
_____
_____
_____
_____

Week 17

From .... to ....

BMR .... Weight .... Goal ....

Day 113		Calories
	Activity	

Day 114		Calories
	Activity	

Day 115		Calories
	Activity	

Day 116		Calories
	Activity	

Day 117		Calories
	Activity	

Day 118		Calories
	Activity	

Day 119		Calories
	Activity	

Week 18

From .... to ....

BMR .... Weight .... Goal ....

Day 120		Calories
	Activity	

Day 121		Calories
	Activity	

Day 122		Calories
	Activity	

Day 123		Calories
	Activity	

Day 124		Calories
	Activity	

Day 125		Calories
	Activity	

Day 126		Calories
	Activity	

Week 19

From .... to ....

BMR .... Weight .... Goal ....

Day 127		Calories
	Activity	

Day 128		Calories
	Activity	

Day 129		Calories
	Activity	

Day 130		Calories
	Activity	

Day 131		Calories
	Activity	

Day 132		Calories
	Activity	

Day 133		Calories
	Activity	

Week 20

From .... to ....

BMR .... Weight .... Goal ....

		Calories
Day 134		
	Activity	

		Calories
Day 135		
	Activity	

		Calories
Day 136		
	Activity	

		Calories
Day 137		
	Activity	

		Calories
Day 138		
	Activity	

		Calories
Day 139		
	Activity	

		Calories
Day 140		
	Activity	

My Recipes

My Recipes

Shopping List

Activities

○

○

○

○

○

Negative Thoughts

Positive Thoughts

○

○

○

○

○

Calorie Record

My BMR is .... kilocalories per day

Day	Date	Morning	Afternoon	Evening	Total
Monday					
Tuesday					
Wednesday					
Thursday					
Friday					
Saturday					
Sunday					

Calorie Record

My BMR is .... kilocalories per day

Day	Date	Morning	Afternoon	Evening	Total
Monday					
Tuesday					
Wednesday					
Thursday					
Friday					
Saturday					
Sunday					

Calorie Record

My BMR is .... kilocalories per day

Day	Date	Morning	Afternoon	Evening	Total
Monday					
Tuesday					
Wednesday					
Thursday					
Friday					
Saturday					
Sunday					

Calorie Record

My BMR is .... kilocalories per day

Day	Date	Morning	Afternoon	Evening	Total
Monday					
Tuesday					
Wednesday					
Thursday					
Friday					
Saturday					
Sunday					

My Goals For Month Six

During the sixth month of my healthy eating plan:

I want to reach my target weight of _____ .

My body mass index is _____ .

My basal metabolic rate is _____ kilocalories per day.

❏　　I reached my target weight last month.

I will continue to exercise at least twice a week, but I am now going to change my exercise plan as follows to keep it fresh:

_____

_____

_____

_____

_____

_____

❏　　I will slightly increase the weights that I use to build up my lean muscle tissue.

❏　　I will learn to cook another 2 tasty low-fat meals.

❏　　I will spend around 30 minutes a day doing a mildly aerobic activity.

❏　　I will reward myself for following my six month plan.

The difficulties I experienced over the six months of my diet plan were:

_____

_____

_____
_____
_____
_____
_____
_____

How I avoided or dealt with these difficulties:

_____
_____
_____
_____
_____
_____
_____

Here is a list of any situations where I wasn't hungry and yet found myself eating:

_____
_____
_____
_____
_____
_____
_____

My goals for the next six months are:

_____
_____
_____
_____
_____
_____
_____

Week 21

From ....   to ....

BMR ....   Weight ....   Goal ....

		Calories
Day 141	Activity	
Day 142	Activity	Calories
Day 143	Activity	Calories
Day 144	Activity	Calories
Day 145	Activity	Calories
Day 146	Activity	Calories
Day 147	Activity	Calories

Week 22

From .... to ....

BMR .... Weight .... Goal ....

		Calories
Day 148		
	Activity	
Day 149		Calories
	Activity	
Day 150		Calories
	Activity	
Day 151		Calories
	Activity	
Day 152		Calories
	Activity	
Day 153		Calories
	Activity	
Day 154		Calories
	Activity	

Week 23

From .... to ....

BMR .... Weight .... Goal ....

Day 155		Calories
	Activity	

Day 156		Calories
	Activity	

Day 157		Calories
	Activity	

Day 158		Calories
	Activity	

Day 159		Calories
	Activity	

Day 160		Calories
	Activity	

Day 161		Calories
	Activity	

Week 24

From .... to ....

BMR .... Weight .... Goal ....

Day 162		Calories
	Activity	

Day 163		Calories
	Activity	

Day 164		Calories
	Activity	

Day 165		Calories
	Activity	

Day 166		Calories
	Activity	

Day 167		Calories
	Activity	

Day 168		Calories
	Activity	

My Recipes

My Recipes

○

○

○

○

○

Shopping List

○

○

○

○

○

Activities

Negative Thoughts

○

○

○

○

○

Positive Thoughts

- O
- O
- O
- O
- O

Calorie Record

My BMR is .... kilocalories per day

Day	Date	Morning	Afternoon	Evening	Total
Monday					
Tuesday					
Wednesday					
Thursday					
Friday					
Saturday					
Sunday					

Calorie Record

My BMR is .... kilocalories per day

Day	Date	Morning	Afternoon	Evening	Total
Monday					
Tuesday					
Wednesday					
Thursday					
Friday					
Saturday					
Sunday					

Calorie Record

My BMR is .... kilocalories per day

Day	Date	Morning	Afternoon	Evening	Total
Monday					
Tuesday					
Wednesday					
Thursday					
Friday					
Saturday					
Sunday					

Calorie Record

My BMR is .... kilocalories per day

Day	Date	Morning	Afternoon	Evening	Total
Monday					
Tuesday					
Wednesday					
Thursday					
Friday					
Saturday					
Sunday					

Calorie Counter

Specific	Amount	Kcals	Carb	Prot	Fat
Fruit					
Apples					
cooking, raw, peeled	100g	35	8.9	0.3	0.1
cooking, stewed with sugar	100g	74	19.1	0.3	0.1
cooking, stewed without sugar	100g	33	8.1	0.3	0.1
eating, raw, without core	100g	47	11.8	0.4	0.1
eating, raw, with core	100g	42	10.5	0.4	0.1
eating, raw, peeled	100g	45	11.2	0.4	0.1
Apricots					
canned in juice	100g	34	8.4	0.5	0.1
canned in syrup	100g	63	16.1	0.4	0.1
raw, without stone	100g	31	8.5	0.3	0.1
semi-dried, ready-to-eat	100g	158	36.5	4.0	0.6
Avocado					
raw, without skin or stone	100g	190	1.9	1.9	19.5
Banana					
with skin	100g	95	23.2	1.2	0.3
Blackberries	100g	62	15.3	0.8	0.2
stewed with sugar	100g	56	13.8	0.7	0.2
stewed without sugar	100g	21	4.4	0.8	0.2
Blackcurrants	100g	28	6.6	0.9	trace
canned in juice	100g	31	7.6	0.8	trace
canned in syrup	100g	72	18.4	0.7	trace
stewed with sugar	100g	58	15.0	0.7	trace
Cherries					
canned in syrup	100g	71	18.5	0.5	trace
cherries, glace	100g	251	66.4	0.4	trace
raw, without stone	100g	48	11.5	0.9	0.1
cherry pie filling	100g	82	21.5	0.4	trace
Clementines					
raw, without skin	100g	37	8.7	0.9	0.1
Currants	100g	267	67.8	2.3	0.4
Damsons					
raw, without stones	100g	34	8.6	0.5	trace
stewed with sugar	100g	74	19.3	0.4	trace
Dates					
dried, with stones	100g	227	57.1	2.8	0.2
raw, with stones	100g	107	26.9	1.3	0.1
Figs					
dried	100g	227	52.9	3.6	1.6
semi-dried, ready-to-eat	100g	209	48.6	3.3	1.5
Fruit pie filling					
average	100g	77	20.1	0.4	trace
Fruit cocktail					
canned in juice	100g	29	7.2	0.4	trace
canned in syrup	100g	57	14.8	0.4	trace
Fruit salad					
home made					
[bananas, oranges,apples, pears and grapes]	100g	55	13.8	0.7	0.1

Specific	Amount	Kcals	Carb	Prot	Fat
Gooseberries	100g	19	3.0	1.1	0.4
dessert, canned in syrup	100g	73	18.5	0.4	0.2
stewed with sugar	100g	54	12.9	0.7	0.3
stewed without sugar	100g	16	2.5	0.9	0.3
Grapefruit					
canned in juice	100g	30	7.3	0.6	trace
canned in syrup	100g	60	15.5	0.5	trace
raw, with skin	100g	20	4.6	0.5	0.1
Grapes					
raw, black and white	100g	60	15.4	0.4	0.1
Kiwi fruit					
raw, without skin	100g	49	10.6	1.1	0.5
Lemons					
raw, with peel	100g	19	3.2	1.0	0.3
Lychees					
canned in syrup	100g	68	17.7	0.4	trace
raw, without stone	100g	58	14.3	0.9	0.1
Mandarin oranges					
canned in juice	100g	32	7.7	0.7	trace
canned in syrup	100g	52	13.4	0.5	trace
Mangoes					
canned in syrup	100g	77	20.3	0.3	trace
raw, without stone or skin	100g	57	14.1	0.7	0.2
Melon					
Canteloupe, without skin or seeds	100g	19	4.2	0.6	0.1
Galia, without skin or seeds	100g	24	5.6	0.5	0.1
Honeydew, without skin or seeds	100g	28	6.6	0.6	0.1
Watermelon, without skin or seeds	100g	31	7.1	0.5	0.3
Mixed fruit					
dried	100g	268	68.1	2.3	0.4
Nectarines					
raw, without stones	100g	40	9.0	1.4	0.1
Olives					
in brine	100g	103	trace	0.9	11.0
Oranges					
raw, without skin	100g	37	8.5	1.1	0.1
Passion fruit					
raw, without skin	100g	36	5.8	2.6	0.4
Paw-paw					
raw	100g	36	8.8	0.5	0.1
Peaches					
canned in juice	100g	39	9.7	0.6	trace
canned in syrup	100g	55	14.0	0.5	trace
raw, without stone	100g	33	7.6	1.0	0.1
Pears					
canned in juice	100g	33	8.5	0.3	trace
canned in syrup	100g	50	13.2	0.2	trace
raw, without core	100g	40	10.0	0.3	0.1
raw, peeled	100g	41	10.4	0.3	0.1
Peel					
mixed, dried	100g	231	59.1	0.3	0.9
Pineapple					
canned in juice	100g	47	12.2	0.3	trace
canned in syrup	100g	64	16.5	0.5	trace
raw, without skin	100g	41	10.1	0.4	0.2

Specific	Amount	Kcals	Carb	Prot	Fat
Plums					
canned in syrup	100g	59	15.5	0.3	trace
raw, without stone	100g	34	8.3	0.5	0.1
stewed with sugar, weighed with stones	100g	75	19.2	0.5	0.1
stewed without sugar, weighed with stones	100g	29	6.9	0.4	0.1
Prunes					
canned in juice	100g	79	19.7	0.7	0.2
canned in syrup	100g	90	23.0	0.6	0.2
semi-dried, ready-to-eat	100g	141	34.0	2.5	0.4
Raisins	100g	272	69.3	2.1	0.4
Raspberries					
canned in syrup	100g	31	7.6	0.5	trace
raw	100g	25	4.6	1.4	0.3
Rhubarb					
canned in syrup	100g	65	16.9	0.5	trace
raw	100g	7	0.8	0.9	0.1
stewed with sugar	100g	48	11.5	0.9	0.1
stewed without sugar	100g	7	0.7	0.9	0.1
Satsumas					
raw, without peel	100g	36	8.5	0.9	0.1
Strawberries					
canned in syrup	100g	65	16.9	0.5	trace
raw	100g	27	6.0	0.8	0.1
Sultanas	100g	275	69.4	2.7	0.4
Tangerines					
raw	100g	35	8.0	0.9	0.1

Vegetables

Specific	Amount	Kcals	Carb	Prot	Fat
Asparagus					
boiled	100g	26	1.4	3.4	0.8
raw	100g	25	2.0	2.9	0.6
Aubergine					
fried in corn oil	100g	302	2.8	1.2	31.9
raw	100g	15	2.2	0.9	0.4
Bamboo Shoots					
canned, drained	100g	39	9.7	0.7	0
Beans					
Aduki, dried, boiled	100g	123	22.5	9.3	0.2
Baked, canned in tomato sauce	100g	84	15.3	5.2	0.6
Baked, canned in tomato sauce, reduced sugar	100g	73	12.5	5.4	0.6
Blackeye, dried, boiled	100g	116	19.9	8.8	0.7
Broad, frozen, boiled	100g	81	11.7	7.9	0.6
Butter beans, canned, re-heated, drained	100g	77	13.0	5.9	0.5
French, frozen, boiled	100g	25	4.7	1.7	0.1
French, raw	100g	24	3.2	1.9	0.5
Mung, dried, boiled	100g	91	15.3	7.6	0.4
Red kidney, canned, re-heated, drained	100g	100	17.8	6.9	0.6
Red kidney, dried, boiled	100g	103	17.4	8.4	0.5
Runner, boiled	100g	186	2.3	1.2	0.5
Runner, raw	100g	22	3.2	1.6	0.4
Soya, dried, boiled	100g	141	5.1	14.0	7.3
Beansprouts					
Mung, stir-fried in blended oil	100g	72	2.5	1.9	6.1
Mung, raw	100g	31	4.0	2.9	0.5

Specific	Amount	Kcals	Carb	Prot	Fat
Beetroot					
boiled	100g	46	9.5	2.3	0.1
pickled, drained	100g	28	5.6	1.2	0.2
raw	100g	36	7.6	1.7	0.1
Black gram					
dried, boiled	100g	89	13.6	7.8	0.4
Broccoli					
boiled	100g	24	1.1	3.1	0.8
raw	100g	33	1.8	4.4	0.9
Brussels sprouts					
boiled	100g	35	3.5	2.9	1.3
frozen, boiled	100g	35	2.5	3.5	1.3
raw	100g	42	4.1	5.3	1.4
Cabbage					
boiled	100g	18	2.5	0.8	0.6
raw	100g	26	4.1	1.7	0.4
white, raw	100g	27	5.0	1.4	0.2
Carrots					
old, boiled	100g	24	4.9	0.6	0.4
old, raw	100g	35	2.5	0.3	0.2
young, boiled	100g	22	4.4	0.6	0.4
young, raw	100g	30	6.0	0.7	0.5
Cauliflower					
boiled	100g	28	2.1	2.9	0.9
raw	100g	34	3.0	3.6	0.9
Celery					
boiled	100g	8	0.8	0.5	0.3
raw	100g	7	0.9	0.5	0.2
Chick peas					
canned, re-heated, drained	100g	115	16.1	7.2	2.9
dried, boiled	100g	121	18.2	8.4	2.1
Chicory					
raw	100g	11	2.8	0.5	0.6
Courgette					
boiled	100g	19	2.0	2.0	0.4
fried in corn oil	100g	63	2.6	2.6	4.8
raw	100g	18	1.8	1.8	0.4
Cucumber					
raw	100g	10	1.5	0.7	0.1
Curly kale					
boiled	100g	24	1.0	2.4	1.1
raw	100g	33	1.4	3.4	1.6
Fennel					
boiled	100g	11	1.5	0.9	0.2
raw	100g	12	1.8	0.9	0.2
Garlic					
raw	100g	98	16.3	7.9	0.6
Gherkins					
pickled, drained	100g	14	2.6	0.9	0.1
Gourd					
raw	100g	11	0.8	1.6	0.2
Hummus	100g	187	11.6	7.6	12.6
Leeks					
boiled	100g	21	2.6	1.2	0.7
raw	100g	22	2.9	1.6	0.5

Specific	Amount	Kcals	Carb	Prot	Fat
Lentils					
green and brown, whole, dried, boiled	100g	105	16.9	8.8	0.7
red, split, dried, boiled	100g	100	17.5	7.6	0.4
Lettuce					
average, raw	100g	14	1.7	0.8	0.5
Iceberg, raw	100g	13	1.9	0.7	0.3
Marrow					
boiled	100g	9	1.6	0.4	0.2
raw	100g	12	2.2	0.5	0.2
Mixed vegetables					
frozen, boiled	100g	42	6.6	3.3	0.5
with chilli, canned	100g	86	9.1	4.3	3.8
Mushrooms					
boiled	100g	11	0.4	1.8	0.3
creamed, canned	100g	80	5.4	3.4	5.0
fried in blended oil	100g	157	0.3	2.4	16.2
fried in butter	100g	157	0.3	2.4	16.2
fried in corn oil	100g	157	0.3	2.4	16.2
raw	100g	135	0.4	1.8	0.5
Mustard and Cress					
raw	100g	13	0.4	1.6	0.6
Okra					
boiled	100g	28	2.7	2.5	0.9
raw	100g	31	3.0	2.8	1.0
stir-fried in corn oil	100g	269	4.4	4.3	26.1
Onions					
boiled	100g	17	3.7	0.6	0.1
cocktail/ silverskin, drained	100g	15	3.1	0.6	0.1
fried in blended oil	100g	164	14.1	2.3	11.2
fried in corn oil	100g	164	14.1	2.3	11.2
fried in lard	100g	164	14.1	2.3	11.2
pickled, drained	100g	24	4.9	0.9	0.2
raw	100g	36	7.9	1.2	0.2
Parsnip					
boiled	100g	66	12.9	1.6	1.2
raw	100g	64	12.5	1.8	1.1
Peas					
boiled	100g	79	10.0	6.7	1.6
canned, re-heated, drained	100g	80	13.5	5.3	0.9
frozen, boiled	100g	69	9.7	6.0	0.9
mange-tout, boiled	100g	261	3.3	3.2	0.1
mange-tout, raw	100g	32	4.2	3.6	0.2
mange-tout, stir-fried in blended oil	100g	71	3.5	3.8	4.8
mushy, canned, re-heated, drained	100g	81	13.8	5.8	0.7
petits pois, frozen, boiled	100g	49	5.5	5.0	0.9
processed, canned, re-heated, drained	100g	99	17.5	6.9	0.7
processed, canned, re-heated, raw	100g	83	11.3	6.9	1.5
Peppers					
capsicum, green, boiled	100g	18	2.6	1.0	0.5
capsicum, green, raw	100g	15	2.6	0.8	0.3
capsicum, red, boiled	100g	34	7.0	1.1	0.4
capsicum, red, raw	100g	32	6.4	1.0	0.4
mixed, raw	100g	20	0.7	2.9	0.6

Specific	Amount	Kcals	Carb	Prot	Fat
Plantain					
boiled	100g	112	28.5	0.8	0.2
fried in vegetable oil	100g	267	47.5	1.5	9.2
raw	100g	117	29.4	1.1	0.3
Potato croquettes					
fried in blended oil	100g	214	21.6	3.7	13.1
Potato powder					
instant, made up with water	100g	57	13.5	1.5	0.1
instant, made up with whole milk	100g	76	14.8	2.4	1.2
Potato waffles (cooked)	100g	842	30.3	3.2	8.2
Potatoes (chips)					
fine cut, frozen, fried in blended oil	100g	364	41.2	4.5	21.3
fine cut, frozen, fried in corn oil	100g	364	41.2	4.5	21.3
fine cut, frozen, fried in dripping	100g	364	41.2	4.5	21.3
homemade, fried in blended oil	100g	189	30.1	3.9	6.7
homemade, fried in corn oil	100g	189	30.1	3.9	6.7
homemade, fried in dripping	100g	189	30.1	3.9	6.7
oven, frozen, baked	100g	162	29.8	3.2	4.2
chip shop, fried in dripping	100g	239	30.5	3.2	12.4
chip shop, fried in blended oil	100g	239	30.5	3.2	12.4
chip shop, fried in vegetable oil	100g	239	30.5	3.2	12.4
straight cut, frozen, fried in blended oil	100g	273	36.0	4.1	13.5
straight cut, frozen, fried in corn oil	100g	273	36.0	4.1	13.5
straight cut, frozen, fried in dripping	100g	273	36.0	4.1	13.5
french fries, retail [burger restaurants]	100g	280	34.0	3.3	15.5
Potatoes (new)					
boiled	100g	75	17.8	1.5	0.3
boiled in skins	100g	66	15.4	1.4	0.3
canned, re-heated, drained	100g	63	15.1	1.5	0.1
raw	100g	70	16.1	1.7	0.3
Potatoes (old)					
baked, flesh and skin	100g	136	31.7	3.9	0.2
baked, flesh only	100g	77	18.0	2.2	0.1
boiled	100g	72	17.0	1.8	0.1
boiled, mashed with butter	100g	104	15.5	1.8	4.3
boiled, mashed with margarine	100g	104	15.5	1.8	4.3
raw	100g	75	17.2	2.1	0.2
roast in blended oil	100g	149	25.9	2.9	4.5
roast in corn oil	100g	149	25.9	2.9	4.5
roast in lard	100g	149	25.9	2.9	4.5
Pumpkin					
raw	100g	13	2.2	0.7	0.2
boiled	100g	13	2.1	0.6	0.3
Quorn	100g	86	2.0	11.8	3.5
Radish					
raw	100g	12	1.9	0.7	0.2
Ratatouille					
canned	100g	38	3.0	1.0	2.5
Spinach					
boiled	100g	19	0.8	2.2	0.8
frozen, boiled	100g	21	0.5	3.1	0.8
raw	100g	25	1.6	2.8	0.8
Spring greens					
boiled	100g	20	1.6	1.9	0.7
raw	100g	33	3.1	3.0	1.0

Specific	Amount	Kcals	Carb	Prot	Fat
Spring onions					
raw	100g	23	3.0	2.0	0.5
Swede					
raw	100g	24	5.0	0.7	0.3
boiled	100g	11	2.3	0.3	0.1
Sweet potato					
boiled	100g	84	20.5	1.1	0.3
raw	100g	87	21.3	1.2	0.3
Sweetcorn					
baby, canned, drained	100g	23	2.0	2.9	0.4
kernels, canned, drained	100g	122	26.6	2.9	1.2
on-the-cob, whole, boiled	100g	66	11.6	2.5	1.4
Tofu					
Soya bean, steamed	100g	73	0.7	8.1	4.2
Soya bean, steamed, fried	100g	261	2.0	23.5	17.7
Tomatoes and tomato-based products					
canned, with juice	100g	16	3.0	1.0	0.1
fried in blended oil	100g	91	5.0	0.7	7.7
fried in corn oil	100g	91	5.0	0.7	7.7
fried in lard	100g	91	5.0	0.7	7.7
grilled	100g	49	8.9	2.0	0.9
passata	100g	29	6.0	1.1	0.2
raw	100g	17	3.1	0.7	0.3
tomato purée	100g	68	12.9	4.5	0.2
Turnip					
boiled	100g	12	2.0	0.6	0.2
raw	100g	23	4.7	0.9	0.3
Watercress					
raw	100g	22	0.4	3.0	1.0
Yam					
boiled	100g	133	33.0	1.7	0.3
raw	100g	114	28.2	1.5	0.3

Nuts

Specific	Amount	Kcals	Carb	Prot	Fat
Almonds	100g	612	6.9	21.1	55.8
Brazil nuts	100g	682	3.1	14.1	68.2
Cashew nuts					
roasted, salted	100g	611	18.8	20.5	50.9
Chestnuts	100g	170	36.6	2.0	2.7
Coconut					
creamed, block	100g	669	7.0	6.0	68.8
dessicated	100g	604	6.4	5.6	62.0
Hazelnuts	100g	650	6.0	14.1	63.5
Macadamia nuts					
salted	100g	748	4.8	7.9	77.6
Mixed nuts	100g	607	7.9	22.9	54.1
Peanuts					
plain	100g	564	12.5	25.6	46.1
roasted, salted	100g	602	7.1	24.5	53.0
dry roasted	100g	589	10.3	25.5	49.8
peanut butter, smooth	100g	623	13.1	22.6	53.7
Pecan nuts	100g	689	5.8	9.2	70.1
Pine nuts	100g	688	4.0	14.0	68.6
Pistachio nuts	100g	331	4.6	9.9	30.5

Specific	Amount	Kcals	Carb	Prot	Fat
Walnuts	100g	688	3.3	14.7	68.5
Nut-based products					
marzipan, home-made	100g	461	50.2	10.4	25.8
marzipan, retail	100g	404	67.6	5.3	14.4
peanut butter, smooth	100g	623	13.1	22.6	53.7
Seeds					
Sesame seeds	100g	578	0.9	18.2	58.0
Sunflower seeds	100g	581	18.6	19.8	47.5
Seed-based products					
Tahini [sesame seed spread]	100g	607	0.9	18.5	58.9

Cereals and Cereal Products

Specific	Amount	Kcals	Carb	Prot	Fat
Biscuits					
Cheddars, mini	100g	534	52.9	11.3	30.2
Cheeselets	100g	464	56.9	10.3	21.7
Chocolate, assorted	100g	524	67.4	5.7	27.6
Club, mint	100g	521	58.9	3.8	30.0
Club, double choc	100g	539	59.3	5.1	29.8
Digestive	100g	499	67.0	6.5	22.1
Digestive with plain chocolate	100g	511	60.8	7.6	26.1
Flapjacks	100g	484	60.4	4.5	26.6
Garibaldis	100g	409	70.5	4.0	9.4
Gingernut	100g	456	79.1	5.6	15.2
Hob nobs	100g	490	65.3	7.1	21.9
Homemade	100g	463	64.3	6.2	21.9
Jaffa cakes	100g	363	67.8	3.5	10.5
Oatcakes	100g	441	63.0	10.0	18.3
Sandwich	100g	513	69.2	5.0	25.9
Semi-sweet	100g	457	74.8	6.7	16.6
Shortbread	100g	498	63.9	5.9	26.1
Short-sweet	100g	469	62.2	6.2	23.4
Wafer, filled	100g	535	66.0	4.7	29.9
Bran					
Wheat	100g	206	26.8	14.1	5.5
Bread					
Brown, average	100g	218	44.3	8.5	2.0
Chapatis, made with fat	100g	328	48.3	8.1	12.8
Chapatis, made without fat	100g	202	43.7	7.3	1.0
Croissants	100g	360	38.3	8.3	20.3
Crumpets, toasted	100g	199	43.4	6.7	1.0
Currant	100g	289	50.7	7.5	7.6
Granary	100g	235	46.3	9.3	2.7
Hovis	100g	212	41.5	9.5	2.0
Malt	100g	268	56.8	8.3	2.4
Naan	100g	336	50.1	8.9	12.5
Pitta	100g	265	57.9	9.2	1.2
Rolls, brown, crusty	100g	255	50.4	10.3	2.8
Rolls, brown, soft	100g	268	51.8	10.0	2.8
Rolls, hamburger buns	100g	264	48.8	9.1	5.0
Rolls, white, crusty	100g	280	57.6	10.9	2.3
Rolls, white, soft	100g	268	51.6	9.2	4.2
Rolls, wholemeal	100g	241	48.3	9.0	2.9
Rye	100g	219	45.8	8.3	1.7

Specific	Amount	Kcals	Carb	Prot	Fat
Vitbe	100g	229	43.4	9.7	3.1
White, 'with added fibre'	100g	230	49.6	7.6	1.5
White, average	100g	235	49.3	8.4	1.9
White, french stick	100g	270	55.4	9.6	2.7
White, fried	100g	503	48.5	7.9	32.2
White, sliced	100g	217	46.8	7.6	1.3
Wholemeal, average	100g	215	41.6	9.2	2.5
Breakfast cereal					
All-Bran	100g	261	46.6	14.0	3.4
Bran Flakes	100g	318	69.3	10.2	1.9
Coco Pops	100g	384	74.0	5.3	1.0
Common Sense Oat Bran Flakes	100g	357	85.9	11.0	4.0
Corn Flakes	100g	360	88.6	7.9	0.7
Crunchy Nut Corn Flakes	100g	398	93.7	7.4	4.0
Frosties	100g	377	93.7	5.3	0.5
Fruit 'n' Fibre	100g	349	72.1	9.0	4.7
Muesli with no added sugar	100g	366	67.1	10.5	7.8
Muesli, Swiss style	100g	363	72.2	9.8	5.9
Oat and Wheat Bran	100g	325	67.7	10.6	3.5
Porridge, with milk	100g	116	13.7	4.8	5.1
Porridge, with water	100g	49	9.0	1.5	1.1
Puffed Wheat	100g	321	67.3	14.2	1.3
Raisin Wheats	100g	337	75.4	9.0	2.0
Ready Brek	100g	373	68.6	11.4	7.8
Rice Krispies	100g	369	89.7	6.1	0.9
Ricicles	100g	381	95.7	4.3	0.5
Shredded Wheat	100g	325	68.3	10.6	3.0
Shreddies	100g	331	74.1	10.1	1.5
Smacks	100g	386	89.6	8.0	2.0
Special K	100g	377	81.7	15.3	1.0
Start	100g	355	81.7	7.9	1.7
Sugar Puffs	100g	348	84.5	5.9	0.8
Sultana Bran	100g	303	67.8	8.5	1.6
Weetabix	100g	352	75.7	11.0	2.7
Weetaflakes	100g	359	79.3	9.2	2.8
Weetos	100g	372	86.1	6.1	2.7
Buns					
Chelsea	100g	366	56.1	7.8	13.8
Currant	100g	296	52.7	7.6	7.5
Hot cross	100g	310	58.5	7.4	6.8
Cakes					
Battenburg	100g	370	50.0	5.9	17.5
Chocolate Krispie, individual	100g	464	73.1	5.6	18.6
Doughnuts, jam	100g	336	48.8	5.7	14.5
Doughnuts, ring	100g	397	47.2	6.1	21.7
Eclairs	100g	396	26.1	5.6	30.6
Fancy Iced, individual	100g	407	68.8	3.8	14.9
Fruit, plain	100g	354	57.9	5.1	12.9
Fruit, rich	100g	341	59.6	3.8	11.0
Fruit, rich, iced	100g	356	62.7	4.1	11.4
Fruit, wholemeal	100g	363	52.8	6.0	15.7
Gateau	100g	337	43.4	5.7	16.8
Madeira	100g	393	58.4	5.4	16.9
Sponge, basic	100g	459	52.4	6.4	26.3
Sponge, fatless	100g	294	53.0	10.1	6.1

Specific	Amount	Kcals	Carb	Prot	Fat
Sponge, jam filled	100g	302	64.2	4.2	4.9
Sponge, butter icing	100g	490	52.4	4.5	30.6
Swiss Rolls, chocolate, individual	100g	337	58.1	4.3	11.3
Teacakes	100g	329	58.3	8.9	8.3
Crackers					
cream	100g	440	68.3	9.5	16.3
wholemeal	100g	413	72.1	10.1	11.3
Crispbread					
rye	100g	321	70.6	9.4	2.1
Custard powder	100g	354	92.0	0.6	0.7
Flour					
chapati brown	100g	333	73.7	11.5	1.2
chapati white	100g	335	77.6	9.8	0.5
cornflour	100g	354	92.0	0.6	0.7
rye flour	100g	335	75.9	8.2	2.0
soya, full fat	100g	447	23.5	36.8	23.5
soya, low-fat	100g	352	28.2	45.3	7.2
wheat , brown	100g	323	68.5	12.6	1.8
wheat, white, breadmaking	100g	341	75.3	11.5	1.4
wheat, white, plain	100g	341	77.7	9.4	1.3
wheat, white, self-raising	100g	330	75.6	8.9	1.2
wheat, wholemeal	100g	310	63.9	12.7	2.2
Noodles					
egg, raw	100g	391	71.7	12.1	8.2
egg, boiled	100g	62	13.0	2.2	0.5
Oatmeal					
raw	100g	375	66.0	11.2	9.2
Pasta					
Macaroni, raw	100g	348	75.8	12.0	1.8
Macaroni, boiled	100g	86	18.5	3.0	0.5
Spaghetti, white, raw	100g	342	74.1	12.0	1.8
Spaghetti, white, boiled	100g	104	22.2	3.6	0.7
Spaghetti, wholemeal, raw	100g	324	66.2	13.4	2.5
Spaghetti, wholemeal, boiled	100g	113	23.2	4.7	0.9
Pancakes					
Scotch	100g	292	43.6	5.8	11.7
Pastries					
Cream horns	100g	435	25.8	3.8	35.8
Custard tarts, individual	100g	277	32.4	6.3	14.5
Danish	100g	374	51.3	5.8	17.6
Eccles cakes	100g	475	59.3	3.9	26.4
Greek	100g	322	40.0	4.7	17.0
Jam tarts	100g	380	62.0	3.3	13.0
Mince pies, individual	100g	423	59.0	4.3	20.4
Flaky, raw	100g	424	34.8	4.2	30.7
Flaky, cooked	100g	560	45.9	5.6	40.6
Shortcrust, raw	100g	449	46.8	5.7	27.9
Shortcrust, cooked	100g	521	54.2	6.6	32.3
Wholemeal, raw	100g	431	38.5	7.7	28.4
Wholemeal, cooked	100g	499	44.6	8.9	32.9
Puddings					
Blackcurrant pie, pastry top and bottom	100g	262	34.5	3.1	13.3
Bread pudding	100g	297	49.7	5.9	9.6
Christmas pudding, home made	100g	291	49.5	4.6	9.7
Crumble, fruit	100g	198	34.0	2.0	6.9

Specific	Amount	Kcals	Carb	Prot	Fat
Crumble, fruit, wholemeal	100g	193	31.7	2.6	7.1
Fruit pie, top crust only	100g	186	28.7	2.0	7.9
Fruit pie, pastry top and bottom	100g	260	34.0	3.0	13.3
Fruit pie, individual	100g	369	56.7	4.3	15.5
Fruit pie, wholemeal, top crust only	100g	183	26.6	2.6	8.1
Fruit pie, wholemeal, pastry top and bottom	100g	251	30.0	4.0	13.6
Lemon meringue pie	100g	319	45.9	4.5	14.4
Pancakes, sweet, made with whole milk	100g	301	35.0	5.9	16.2
Pie, with pie filling	100g	273	34.6	3.2	14.5
Sponge pudding	100g	340	45.3	5.8	16.3
Treacle tart	100g	368	60.4	3.7	14.1
Rice					
brown, raw	100g	357	81.3	6.7	2.8
brown, boiled	100g	141	32.1	2.6	1.1
savoury, raw	100g	415	77.4	8.4	10.3
savoury, cooked	100g	142	26.3	2.9	3.5
white, easy cook, raw	100g	383	85.8	7.3	3.6
white, easy cook, boiled	100g	138	30.9	2.6	1.3
white, fried in lard	100g	131	25.0	2.2	3.2
Sago					
raw	100g	355	94.0	0.2	0.2
Savouries					
Cauliflower cheese	100g	105	5.1	5.9	6.9
Dumplings	100g	208	24.5	2.8	11.7
Macaroni cheese	100g	178	13.6	7.3	10.8
Pancakes, savoury, made with whole milk	100g	273	24.0	6.3	17.5
Ravioli, in tomato sauce	100g	70	10.3	3.0	2.2
Risotto, plain	100g	224	34.4	3.0	9.3
Samosas, meat	100g	593	17.9	5.1	56.1
Samosas, vegetable	100g	472	22.3	3.1	41.8
Spaghetti, canned in tomato sauce	100g	64	14.1	1.9	0.4
Stuffing, sage and onion	100g	231	20.4	5.2	14.8
Stuffing mix	100g	338	67.2	9.9	5.2
Stuffing mix, made with water	100g	97	19.3	2.8	1.5
Yorkshire pudding	100g	208	24.7	6.6	9.9
Scones					
fruit	100g	316	52.9	7.3	9.8
plain	100g	362	53.8	7.2	14.6
wholemeal	100g	326	43.1	5.8	11.7
Tapioca					
raw	100g	359	95.0	0.4	0.1
Wheatgerm	100g	357	44.7	26.7	9.2

Milk and Dairy Produce

	Amount	Kcals	Carb	Prot	Fat
Butter	100g	737	trace	0.5	81.7
Cheese					
Brie	100g	319	trace	19.3	26.9
Camembert	100g	297	trace	20.9	23.7
Cheddar, average	100g	412	0.1	25.5	34.4
Cheddar, vegetarian	100g	425	trace	25.8	35.7
Cheddar-type, reduced fat	100g	261	trace	31.5	15.0
Cheese spread	100g	276	4.4	13.5	22.8
Cottage cheese, plain	100g	98	2.1	13.8	3.9
Cottage cheese, reduced fat	100g	78	3.3	13.3	1.4

Specific	Amount	Kcals	Carb	Prot	Fat
Cottage cheese, with additions	100g	95	2.6	12.8	3.8
Cream cheese	100g	439	trace	3.1	47.4
Danish blue	100g	347	trace	20.1	29.6
Edam	100g	333	trace	26.0	25.4
Feta	100g	250	1.5	15.6	20.2
Fromage frais, fruit	100g	131	13.8	6.8	5.8
Fromage frais, plain	100g	113	5.7	6.8	7.1
Fromage frais, very low-fat	100g	58	6.8	7.7	0.2
Gouda	100g	375	trace	24.0	31.0
Hard cheese, average	100g	405	0.1	24.7	34.0
Parmesan	100g	452	trace	39.4	32.7
Parmesan	10g portion	45	trace	3.9	3.3
Processed, plain	100g	330	0.9	20.8	27.0
Soft cheese, full fat	100g	313	trace	8.6	31.0
Soft cheese, medium fat	100g	179	3.1	9.2	14.5
Stilton	100g	411	0.1	22.7	35.5
White, average	100g	376	0.1	23.4	31.3
Cream, fresh					
clotted	100g	586	2.3	1.6	63.5
double	100g	449	2.7	1.7	48.0
half	100g	148	4.3	3.0	13.3
single	100g	198	4.1	2.6	19.1
soured	100g	205	3.8	2.9	19.9
whipping	100g	373	3.1	2.0	39.3
Cream, imitation					
Dessert Top	100g	291	6.0	2.4	28.8
Dream Topping, made with semi-skimmed milk	100g	166	12.2	3.9	11.7
Dream Topping, made with whole milk	100g	182	12.1	3.8	13.5
Elmlea, double	100g	454	3.2	2.5	48.0
Elmlea, single	100g	190	4.1	3.2	18.0
Elmlea, whipping	100g	319	3.2	2.5	33.0
Tip Top	100g	110	8.5	5.0	6.5
Cream, sterilised					
canned	100g	239	3.7	2.5	23.9
Cream, uht					
canned spray	100g	309	3.5	1.9	32.0
Dairy/fat spread	100g	662	trace	0.4	73.4
Dessert					
Cheesecake	100g	242	33.0	5.7	10.6
Custard, made with skimmed milk	100g	79	16.8	3.8	0.1
Custard, made with whole milk	100g	117	16.6	3.7	4.5
Instant dessert, made with skimmed milk	100g	97	14.9	3.1	3.2
Instant dessert, made with whole milk	100g	125	14.8	3.1	6.3
Milk pudding, made with skimmed milk	100g	93	20.1	4.0	0.2
Milk pudding, made with whole milk	100g	129	19.9	3.9	4.3
Mousse, chocolate	100g	139	19.9	4.0	5.4
Mousse, fruit	100g	137	18.0	4.5	5.7
Rice pudding, canned	100g	89	14.0	3.4	2.5
Trifle, home-made	100g	160	22.3	3.6	6.3
Trifle, home-made, with fresh cream	100g	166	19.5	2.4	9.2
Ice cream					
Choc ice	100g	277	28.1	3.5	17.5
Cornetto	100g	260	34.5	3.7	12.9
Dairy, flavoured	100g	179	24.7	3.5	8.0
Dairy, vanilla	100g	194	24.4	3.6	9.8

Specific	Amount	Kcals	Carb	Prot	Fat
Lemon sorbet	100g	131	34.2	0.9	trace
Non-dairy, flavoured	100g	166	23.2	3.1	7.4
Non-dairy, vanilla	100g	178	23.1	3.2	8.7
Ice cream dessert					
Arctic roll	100g	200	33.3	4.1	6.6
assorted, average	100g	227	22.8	3.3	14.2
Chocolate nut sundae	100g	278	34.2	3.0	15.3
Ice cream mix, prepared	100g	182	25.1	4.1	7.9
Milk, condensed					
skimmed, sweetened	100g	267	60.0	10.0	0.2
whole, sweetened	100g	333	55.5	8.5	10.1
Milk, dried skimmed	100g	348	52.9	36.1	0.6
skimmed, with vegetable fat	100g	487	42.6	23.3	25.9
Milk, evaporated					
whole	100g	151	8.5	8.4	9.4
Milk, flavoured					
mixed flavours, skimmed	100g	68	10.6	3.6	1.5
Milk, goat's					
pasteurised	100g	60	4.4	3.1	3.5
Milk, semi-skimmed					
pasteurised	100g	46	5.0	3.3	1.6
fortified plus smp	100g	51	5.8	3.7	1.6
UHT	100g	46	4.8	3.3	1.7
Milk, sheep's					
raw	100g	95	5.1	5.4	6.0
pasteurised	100g	33	5.0	3.3	0.1
Milk, skimmed					
pasteurised	100g	33	5.0	3.3	trace
fortified plus smp	100g	39	6.0	3.8	0.1
UHT fortified	100g	35	5.0	3.5	0.2
Milk, soya alternative					
plain	100g	32	0.8	2.9	1.9
flavoured	100g	40	3.6	2.8	1.7
Milk, whole					
pasteurised	100g	66	4.8	3.2	3.9
sterilised	100g	66	4.5	3.5	3.9
UHT, fortified	100g	35	5.0	3.5	0.2
Yoghurt					
drinking	100g	62	13.1	3.1	trace
Greek, cow's	100g	115	2.0	6.4	9.1
Greek, sheep's	100g	106	5.6	4.4	7.5
low-calorie	100g	41	6.0	4.3	0.2
low-fat, flavoured	100g	90	17.9	3.8	0.9
low-fat, fruit	100g	90	17.9	4.1	0.7
low-fat, plain	100g	56	7.5	5.1	0.8
soya alternative	100g	72	3.9	5.0	4.2
whole milk, fruit	100g	105	15.7	5.1	2.8
whole milk, plain	100g	79	7.8	5.7	3.0
Yoghurt-based dish					
Tzatziki	100g	66	2.0	3.7	4.9

Eggs and Egg-based Products

	Amount	Kcals	Carb	Prot	Fat
Chicken's egg					
boiled	100g	147	trace	12.5	10.8

Specific	Amount	Kcals	Carb	Prot	Fat
boiled	1, size 1 [67g]	98	trace	8.4	7.2
boiled	1, size 2 [61g]	90	trace	7.6	6.6
boiled	1, size 3 [57g]	84	trace	7.1	6.2
boiled	1, size 4 [47g]	69	trace	5.9	5.1
fried in vegetable oil	100g	179	trace	13.6	13.9
fried in vegetable oil	1, average [60g]	107	trace	8.2	8.3
poached	100g	147	trace	12.5	10.8
poached	1, average [50g]	74	trace	6.3	5.4
scrambled, with milk	100g	247	0.6	10.7	22.6
white, raw	100g	36	trace	9.0	trace
whole, raw	100g	147	trace	12.5	10.8
whole, raw	1, size 1 [67g]	98	trace	8.4	7.2
whole, raw	1, size 2 [61g]	90	trace	7.6	6.6
whole, raw	1, size 3 [57g]	84	trace	7.1	6.2
whole, raw	1, size 4 [47g]	69	trace	5.9	5.1
yolk, raw	100g	339	trace	16.1	30.5
Duck egg					
whole, raw	100g	163	trace	14.3	11.8
whole, raw	1, average [75g]	122	trace	17.2	14.2
Egg-based dessert					
Meringue, with cream	100g	376	40.0	3.3	23.6
Meringue, without cream	100g	379	95.4	5.3	trace
Egg-based dish					
Egg fried rice	100g	208	25.7	4.2	10.6
Omelette, cheese	100g	266	trace	15.9	22.6
Omelette, plain	100g	191	trace	10.9	16.4
Quiche, cheese and egg	100g	314	17.3	12.5	22.2
Quiche, cheese and egg, wholemeal	100g	308	14.5	13.2	22.4
Scotch egg	100g	251	13.1	12.0	17.1

Meat and Meat Products

Specific	Amount	Kcals	Carb	Prot	Fat
Bacon					
Gammon joint, boiled	100g	269	0	24.7	18.9
Gammon joint, raw	100g	236	0	17.6	18.3
Gammon rasher, grilled	100g	228	0	29.5	12.2
Rasher [back], grilled	100g	405	0	25.3	33.8
Rasher [back], raw	100g	428	0	14.2	41.2
Rasher [middle], grilled	100g	416	0	24.9	35.1
Rasher [middle], raw	100g	425	0	14.3	40.9
Rasher [streaky], grilled	100g	422	0	24.5	36.0
Rasher [streaky], raw	100g	414	0	14.6	39.5
Beef					
Brisket, boiled	100g	326	0	27.6	23.9
Brisket, boiled	200g portion	652	0	55.2	47.8
Brisket, raw	100g	252	0	16.8	20.5
Mince, raw	100g	221	0	18.8	16.2
Mince, stewed	100g	229	0	23.1	15.2
Rump steak, fried	100g	246	0	28.6	14.6
Rump steak, grilled	100g	218	0	27.3	12.1
Rump steak, raw	100g	197	0	18.9	13.5
salted	100g	119	0	27.1	0.4
Silverside, salted, boiled	100g	242	0	28.6	14.2
Sirloin, raw	100g	272	0	16.6	22.8
Sirloin, roast	100g	284	0	23.6	21.1

Specific	Amount	Kcals	Carb	Prot	Fat
Stewing steak, raw	100g	176	0	20.2	10.6
Stewing steak, stewed	100g	223	0	30.9	11.0
Topside, raw	100g	179	0	19.6	11.2
Topside, roast	100g	214	0	26.6	12.0
Beef-based dish					
Beef kheema	100g	413	0.3	18.2	37.7
Beef steak pudding	100g	224	18.8	10.8	12.3
Beef stew, home made	100g	120	4.6	9.7	7.2
Bolognese sauce	100g	145	3.7	8.0	11.1
Chilli con carne	100g	151	8.3	11.0	8.5
Chow mein	100g	136	14.7	6.7	6.0
Curry	100g	137	6.3	13.5	6.6
Curry with rice	100g	137	16.9	8.8	4.3
Stewed steak, canned, with gravy	100g	176	1.0	14.8	12.5
Beefburgers, frozen, raw	100g	265	5.3	15.2	20.5
Beefburgers, frozen, fried	100g	264	7.0	20.4	17.3
Corned beef, canned	100g	217	0	26.9	12.1
Chicken and chicken-based dishes					
Breaded, fried in oil	100g	242	14.8	18.0	12.7
Dark meat, boiled	100g	204	0	28.6	9.9
Dark meat, raw	100g	126	0	19.1	5.5
Dark meat, roast	100g	155	0	23.1	6.9
Leg quarter, roast	100g	92	0	15.4	3.4
Light and dark meat, boiled	100g	183	0	29.2	7.3
Light and dark meat, raw	100g	121	0	20.5	4.3
Light and dark meat, roast	100g	148	0	24.8	5.4
Light meat, boiled	100g	163	0	29.7	4.9
Light meat, raw	100g	116	0	21.8	3.2
Light meat, roast	100g	142	0	26.5	4.0
Wing quarter, roast	100g	74	0	12.4	2.7
Chicken in white sauce, canned	100g	176	3.5	9.5	15.0
Curry	100g	205	3.1	10.2	17.0
Curry with rice	100g	144	16.9	7.8	5.5
Duck					
roast	100g	189	0	25.3	9.7
Goose					
roast	100g	319	0	29.3	22.4
Grouse					
roast	100g	173	0	31.3	5.3
Ham					
canned	100g	120	0	18.4	5.1
honey roast	100g	108	2.4	18.2	2.9
smoked	100g	94	0.8	17.6	2.3
Hare					
stewed	100g	192	0	29.9	8.0
Lamb and lamb dishes					
breast, raw	100g	378	0	16.7	34.6
breast, roast	100g	410	0	19.1	37.1
chops, loin, grilled	100g	355	0	23.5	29.0
chops, loin, raw	100g	377	0	14.6	35.4
cutlets, grilled	100g	370	0	23.0	30.9
cutlets, raw	100g	386	0	14.7	36.3
leg, raw	100g	240	0	17.9	18.7
leg, roast	100g	266	0	26.1	17.9
scrag and neck, raw	100g	316	0	15.6	28.2

Specific	Amount	Kcals	Carb	Prot	Fat
Scrag and neck, stewed	100g	292	0	25.6	21.1
Shoulder, raw	100g	314	0	15.6	28.0
Shoulder, roast	100g	316	0	19.9	26.3
Irish stew	100g	123	9.1	5.3	7.6
Lamb kheema	100g	328	2.3	14.6	29.1
Moussaka	100g	184	7.0	9.1	13.6
Lamb hot pot, frozen	100g	92	7.9	7.9	3.4
Moussaka, frozen	100g	105	9.9	7.0	4.4
Meat-based dish					
Cottage pie, frozen	100g	110	11.4	5.1	4.7
Hot pot, home made	100g	114	10.1	9.4	4.5
Lasagne	100g	102	12.8	5.0	3.8
Meat curry	100g	162	9.1	8.5	10.5
Shepherd's pie	100g	118	8.2	8.0	6.2
Meat-based products					
Black pudding, fried	100g	305	15.0	12.9	21.9
Brawn	100g	153	0	12.4	11.5
Chopped ham and pork, canned	100g	275	1.4	14.4	23.6
Cornish pasty	100g	332	31.1	8.0	20.4
Faggots	100g	268	15.3	11.1	18.5
Frankfurters	100g	274	3.0	9.5	25.0
Grillsteaks, grilled	100g	305	0.5	22.1	23.9
Haggis, boiled	100g	310	19.2	10.7	21.7
Liver pâté	100g	316	1.0	13.1	28.9
Liver pâté, low-fat	100g	191	2.8	18.0	12.0
Liver sausage	100g	310	4.3	12.9	26.9
Luncheon meat, canned	100g	313	5.5	12.6	26.9
Meat paste	100g	173	3.0	15.2	11.2
Pepperami	100g	560	1.0	20	52
Polony	100g	281	14.2	9.4	21.1
Pork pie, individual	100g	376	24.9	9.8	27.0
Salami	100g	491	1.9	19.3	45.2
Sausage roll, flaky pastry	100g	477	32.3	7.1	36.4
Sausage roll, short pastry	100g	459	37.5	8.0	31.9
Saveloy	100g	262	10.1	9.9	20.5
Steak and kidney pie, individual, pastry top and bottom	100g	323	25.6	9.1	21.2
Steak and kidney pie, pastry top only	100g	286	15.9	15.2	18.4
White pudding	100g	450	36.3	7.0	31.8
Sausages, beef, fried	100g	269	14.9	12.9	18.0
Sausages, beef, grilled	100g	265	15.2	13.0	17.3
Sausages, beef, raw	100g	299	11.7	9.6	24.1
Sausages, pork, fried	100g	317	11.0	13.8	24.5
Sausages, pork, grilled	100g	318	11.5	13.3	24.6
Sausages, pork, low-fat, fried	100g	211	9.1	14.9	13.0
Sausages, pork, low-fat, grilled	100g	229	10.8	16.2	13.8
Sausages, pork, low-fat, raw	100g	166	8.1	12.5	9.5
Sausages, pork, raw	100g	367	9.5	10.6	32.1
Offal					
Heart, lamb, raw	100g	119	0	17.1	5.6
Heart, ox, raw	100g	108	0	18.9	3.6
Heart, ox, stewed	100g	179	0	31.4	5.9
Heart, sheep, roast	100g	237	0	26.1	14.7
Kidney, lamb, fried	100g	155	0	24.6	6.3
Kidney, lamb,raw	100g	90	0	16.5	2.7
Kidney, ox, raw	100g	86	0	15.7	2.6

Specific	Amount	Kcals	Carb	Prot	Fat
Kidney, ox, stewed	100g	172	0	25.6	7.7
Kidney, pig, raw	100g	90	0	16.3	2.7
Kidney, pig, stewed	100g	153	0	24.4	6.1
Liver, calf, coated in flour and fried	100g	254	7.3	26.9	13.2
Liver, calf, raw	100g	153	1.9	20.1	7.3
Liver, chicken, coated in flour and fried	100g	194	3.4	20.7	10.9
Liver, chicken, raw	100g	135	0.6	19.1	6.3
Liver, lamb, coated in flour and fried	100g	232	3.9	22.9	14.0
Liver, lamb, raw	100g	179	1.6	20.1	10.3
Liver, ox raw	100g	163	2.2	21.1	7.8
Liver, ox, coated in flour and stewed	100g	198	3.6	24.8	9.5
Liver, pig, coated in flour and stewed	100g	189	3.6	25.6	8.1
Liver, pig, raw	100g	154	2.1	21.3	6.8
Oxtail, stewed	100g	243	0	30.5	13.4
Sweetbread, lamb, in egg and breadcrumbs and fried	100g	230	5.6	19.4	14.6
Sweetbread, lamb, raw	100g	131	0	15.3	7.8
Tongue, lamb, raw	100g	193	0	15.3	14.6
Tongue, ox, boiled	100g	293	0	19.5	23.9
Tongue, ox, pickled, raw	100g	220	0	15.7	17.5
Tongue, sheep, stewed	100g	289	0	18.2	24.0
Partridge					
roast	100g	212	0	36.7	7.2
Pheasant					
roast	100g	213	0	32.2	9.3
Pigeon					
roast	100g	230	0	27.8	13.2
Pork					
belly rashers, grilled	100g	398	0	21.1	34.8
belly rashers, raw	100g	381	0	15.3	35.5
chops, loin, grilled	100g	332	0	28.5	24.2
chops, loin, raw	100g	329	0	15.9	29.5
leg, raw	100g	269	0	16.6	22.5
leg, roast	100g	286	0	26.9	19.8
trotters and tails, boiled	100g	280	0	19.8	22.3
Rabbit					
raw	100g	124	0	21.9	4.0
stewed	100g	179	0	27.3	7.7
Tongue					
canned	100g	213	0	16.0	16.5
Turkey and turkey-based products					
dark meat, raw	100g	114	0	20.3	3.6
dark meat, roast	100g	148	0	27.8	4.1
light and dark meat, raw	100g	107	0	21.9	2.2
light and dark meat, roast	100g	140	0	28.8	2.7
light meat, raw	100g	103	0	23.2	1.1
light meat, roast	100g	132	0	29.8	1.4
Turkey with ham	100g	123	2.2	19.2	4.1
Veal					
cutlet, coated in egg and breadcrumbs and fried	100g	215	4.4	31.4	8.1
fillet, raw	100g	109	0	21.1	2.7
fillet, roast	100g	230	0	31.6	11.5
Venison					
haunch, roast	100g	198	0	35.0	6.4

Specific	Amount	Kcals	Carb	Prot	Fat
		Fish and Seafood			
Anchovies					
canned in oil, drained	100g	280	0	25.2	19.9
Cockles					
boiled	100g	48	trace	11.3	0.3
Cod					
dried, salted, boiled	100g	138	0	32.5	0.9
fillets, baked, with butter added	100g	96	0	21.4	1.2
fillets, poached in milk with butter added	100g	94	0	20.9	1.1
fillets, raw	100g	76	0	17.4	0.7
in batter, fried in blended oil	100g	199	7.5	19.6	10.3
in batter, fried in dripping	100g	199	7.5	19.6	10.3
steaks, frozen, raw,	100g	68	0	15.6	0.6
Crab					
boiled	100g	127	0	20.1	5.2
canned	100g	81	0	18.1	0.9
Dogfish					
in batter, fried in blended oil	100g	265	7.7	16.7	18.8
in batter, fried in dripping	100g	265	7.7	16.7	18.8
Fish fingers					
fried in blended oil	100g	233	17.2	13.5	12.7
grilled	100g	214	19.3	15.1	9.0
Fish-based dish					
Fish pie, home-made	100g	105	12.3	8.0	3.0
Kedgeree, home-made	100g	166	10.5	14.2	7.9
Fish-based product					
Fish cakes, fried	100g	188	15.1	9.1	10.5
Fish paste	100g	169	3.7	15.3	10.4
Taramasalata	100g	446	4.1	3.2	46.4
Haddock					
fillet, raw	100g	73	0	16.8	0.6
in breadcrumbs, fried in blended oil	100g	174	3.6	21.4	8.3
in breadcrumbs, fried in dripping	100g	174	3.6	21.4	8.3
middle cut, steamed	100g	98	0	22.8	0.8
smoked, steamed	100g	101	0	23.3	0.9
middle cut, steamed	100g	98	0	22.8	0.8
Halibut					
middle cut, steamed	100g	98	0	22.8	0.8
raw	100g	92	0	17.7	2.4
Herring					
fried in oatmeal	100g	234	1.5	23.1	15.1
grilled	100g	135	0	13.9	8.8
raw	100g	234	0	16.8	18.5
Kipper					
baked	100g	205	0	25.5	11.4
Lemon sole					
in breadcrumbs, fried	100g	216	9.3	16.1	13.0
raw	100g	81	0	17.1	1.4
steamed	100g	91	0	20.6	0.9
Lobster					
boiled	100g	119	0	22.1	3.4
Mackerel					
fried	100g	188	0	21.5	11.3
raw	100g	223	0	19.0	16.3
smoked	100g	354	0	18.9	30.9

Specific	Amount	Kcals	Carb	Prot	Fat
Mussels					
boiled	100g	87	trace	17.2	2.0
Pilchards					
in tomato sauce, canned	100g	126	0.7	18.8	5.4
in batter, fried in dripping	100g	279	14.4	15.8	18.0
in breadcrumbs, fried	100g	228	8.6	18.0	13.7
raw	100g	91	0	17.9	2.2
steamed	100g	93	0	18.9	1.9
Prawns					
boiled	100g	107	0	22.6	1.8
Roe					
Cod, hard, in breadcrumbs, fried	100g	202	3.0	20.9	11.9
Herring, soft, rolled in flour and fried	100g	244	4.7	21.1	15.8
Saithe					
raw	100g	73	0	17.0	0.5
steamed	100g	99	0	23.3	0.6
Salmon					
canned	100g	155	0	20.3	8.2
raw	100g	182	0	18.4	12.0
smoked	100g	142	0	25.4	4.5
steamed	100g	197	0	20.1	13.0
Sardines					
in oil, canned, drained	100g	217	0	23.7	13.6
in tomato sauce, canned	100g	177	0.5	17.8	11.6
Scampi					
in breadcrumbs, fried	100g	316	28.9	12.2	17.6
Shrimps					
canned, drained	100g	94	0	20.8	1.2
frozen	100g	73	0	16.5	0.8
Skate					
in batter, fried	100g	199	4.9	17.9	12.1
Squid					
frozen, raw	100g	66	0	13.1	1.5
Trout					
brown, steamed	100g	135	0	23.5	4.5
Tuna					
in brine, canned, drained	100g	99	0	23.5	0.6
in oil, canned, drained	100g	189	0	27.1	9.0
Whelks					
boiled, weighed with shell	100g	14	trace	2.8	0.3
Whitebait					
rolled in flour, fried	100g	525	5.3	19.5	47.5
Whiting					
in breadcrumbs, fried	100g	191	7.0	18.1	10.3
steamed	100g	92	0	20.9	0.9
Winkles					
boiled, weighed with shell	100g	14	trace	2.9	0.3

Desserts

Specific	Amount	Kcals	Carb	Prot	Fat
Blackcurrant pie					
home-made, pastry top and bottom	100g	262	34.5	3.1	13.3
Bread pudding					
home-made	100g	297	49.7	5.9	9.6
Cheesecake					
frozen, with fruit	100g	242	33.0	5.7	10.6

Specific	Amount	Kcals	Carb	Prot	Fat
individual, fruit purée topping	100g	274	32.4	5.8	13.5
Christmas pudding					
home-made	100g [average portion]	291	49.5	4.6	9.7
retail	100g [average portion]	329	56.3	3.0	11.8
Creamed rice					
canned	100g	91	15.2	3.4	1.8
Creamed sago					
canned	100g	82	13.0	2.9	1.8
Creamed semolina					
canned	100g	84	13.2	3.6	1.9
Creme caramel					
individual	100g	109	20.6	3.0	2.2
Custard					
chocolate-flavoured, powdered	100g, powder only	409	82.0	6.0	9.0
home-made, made with skimmed milk	100g	79	16.8	3.8	0.1
home-made, made with whole milk	100g	117	16.6	3.7	4.5
low-fat, canned	100g	75	12.5	3.0	1.4
Dessert topping					
Evaporated milk	100g	159	12.0	8.2	9.0
Tip Top	100g	112	9.0	4.8	6.3
Frozen dessert					
Arctic roll	100g	200	33.3	4.1	6.6
Chocolate nut sundae, individual	100g	278	34.2	3.0	15.3
Viennetta	100g	272	27.6	3.8	16.4
Frozen ice cream dessert, average	100g	227	22.8	3.3	14.2
Fruit crumble					
home-made	100g	198	34.0	2.0	6.9
wholemeal, home-made	100g	193	31.7	2.6	7.1
Fruit pie					
pastry top and bottom	100g	262	34.5	3.1	13.3
Fruit pie filling					
apple and blackberry, canned	100g	92	24.1	0.3	trace
black cherry, canned	100g	98	25.8	0.3	trace
Ice cream					
choc ice	100g	277	28.1	3.5	17.5
Cornetto	100g	260	34.5	3.7	12.9
dairy, vanilla	100g	194	24.4	3.6	9.8
flavoured	100g	179	24.7	3.5	8.0
non-dairy, flavoured	100g	166	23.2	3.1	7.4
non-dairy, vanilla	100g	178	23.1	3.2	8.7
ice cream mix	100g	182	25.1	4.1	7.9
ice cream wafers	100g	342	78.8	10.1	0.7
Instant dessert powder					
Angel delight	100g, powder only	468	73.8	2.3	19.0
Average, made with whole milk	100g	125	14.8	3.1	6.3
Average, made with skimmed milk	100g	97	14.9	3.1	3.2
Jelly					
Fruit-flavoured, before dilution	100g	280	69.7	4.7	trace
Lemon meringue pie					
Home-made	100g	319	45.9	4.5	14.4
Meringue					
home-made	100g	379	95.4	5.3	trace
home-made, with cream	100g	376	40.0	3.3	23.6
Mousse					
chocolate, individual	100g	139	19.9	4.0	5.4

Specific	Amount	Kcals	Carb	Prot	Fat
fruit, individual	100g	137	18.0	4.5	5.7
Pancakes					
sweet, made with whole milk	100g	301	35.0	5.9	16.2
Pie					
with pie filling	100g	273	34.6	3.2	14.5
Rice Pudding					
average, canned	100g	89	14.0	3.4	2.5
traditional, with sultanas and nutmeg	100g	101	17.1	3.3	2.6
Sorbet					
lemon, home-made	100g	131	34.2	0.9	trace
Sponge pudding					
home-made	100g	340	45.3	5.8	16.3
Steamed sponge pudding					
chocolate, with chocolate sauce, canned	100g	299	51.2	2.6	9.3
treacle, canned	100g	301	51.4	2.2	9.6
with jam, canned	100g	299	49.8	2.6	9.9
Trifle					
fruit cocktail, individual	100g	182	23.1	2.5	2.6
home-made	100g	160	22.3	3.6	6.3
home-made, with cream	100g	166	19.5	2.4	9.2
milk chocolate, individual	100g	282	25.1	4.7	18.2
raspberry, individual	100g	173	21.1	2.5	8.7
Yoghurt					
Greek, strained	100g	115	2.0	6.4	9.1
low-fat, fruit	100g	90	17.9	4.1	0.7
low-fat, plain	100g	56	7.5	5.1	0.8
very low-fat, fruit	100g	45	6.3	5.2	0.1
whole milk, fruit	100g	105	15.7	5.1	2.8
whole milk, plain	100g	79	7.8	5.7	3.0

Sauces, Soup and Miscellaneous

Specific	Amount	Kcals	Carb	Prot	Fat
Chutney					
apple	100g	201	52.2	0.9	0.2
mango	100g	285	49.5	0.4	10.9
tomato	100g	161	40.9	1.2	0.4
Miscellaneous					
Baking powder	100g	163	37.8	5.2	trace
Bovril	100g	169	2.9	38.0	0.7
Gelatine	100g	338	0	84	0
Gravy granules, made with water	100g	462	40.6	4.4	32.5
Marmite	100g	172	1.8	39.7	0.7
Mustard, smooth	100g	139	9.7	7.1	8.2
Mustard, wholegrain	100g	140	4.2	8.2	10.2
Oxo cubes	100g	229	12.0	38.3	3.4
Salt	100g	0	0	0	0
Vinegar	100g	4	0.6	0.4	0
Yeast, baker's compressed	100g	5	1.1	11.4	0.4
Yeast, dried	100g	169	3.5	35.6	1.5
Pickle					
sweet	100g	134	34.4	0.6	0.3
Salad dressing					
French dressing	100g	649	0.1	0.3	72.1
Mayonnaise	100g	691	1.7	1.1	75.6
Salad cream	100g	348	16.7	1.5	31.0

Specific	Amount	Kcals	Carb	Prot	Fat
Salad cream, reduced calorie	100g	194	9.4	1.0	17.2
Sauce					
Barbecue	100g	75	12.2	1.8	1.8
Bread sauce, made with semi-skimmed milk	100g	93	12.8	4.3	3.1
Bread sauce, made with whole milk	100g	110	12.6	4.2	5.1
Brown sauce, bottled	100g	99	25.2	1.1	0
Cheese sauce, made with semi-skimmed milk	100g	179	9.1	8.1	12.6
Cheese sauce, made with whole milk	100g	197	9.0	8.0	14.6
Cheese sauce, packet mix, made with semi-skimmed milk	100g	90	9.5	5.4	3.8
Cheese sauce, packet mix, made with whole milk	100g	110	9.3	5.3	6.1
Cook-in sauces, canned, average	100g	43	8.3	1.1	0.8
Curry sauce, canned	100g	78	7.1	1.5	5.0
Horseradish sauce	100g	153	17.9	2.5	8.4
Mint sauce	100g	87	21.5	1.6	trace
Onion sauce, made with semi-skimmed milk	100g	86	8.4	2.9	5.0
Onion sauce, made with whole milk	100g	99	8.3	2.8	6.5
Pasta sauce, tomato based	100g	47	6.9	2.0	1.5
Soy sauce	100g	64	8.3	8.7	0
Tomato ketchup	100g	98	24.0	2.1	trace
Tomato sauce, home-made	100g	89	8.6	2.2	5.5
White sauce, savoury, made with semi-skimmed milk	100g	128	11.1	4.2	7.8
White sauce, savoury, made with whole milk	100g	150	10.9	4.1	10.3
White sauce, sweet, made with semi-skimmed milk	100g	150	18.8	3.9	7.2
White sauce, sweet, made with whole milk	100g	170	18.6	3.8	9.5
Soup					
Chicken noodle, dried, cooked	100g	20	3.7	0.8	0.3
Cream of chicken, canned	100g	58	4.5	1.7	3.8
Cream of chicken, condensed, canned	100g	98	6.0	2.6	7.2
Cream of chicken, condensed, diluted	100g	49	3.0	1.3	3.6
Cream of mushroom soup, canned	100g	53	3.9	1.1	3.8
Cream of tomato, canned	100g	55	5.9	0.8	3.3
Cream of tomato, condensed, canned	100g	123	14.6	1.7	6.8
Cream of tomato, condensed, diluted	100g	62	7.3	0.9	3.4
Instant soup powder, made with water, cooked	100g	64	10.5	1.1	2.3
Lentil, home-made	100g	99	12.7	4.4	3.8
Low-calorie, average, canned	100g	20	4.0	0.9	0.2
Minestrone, dried, cooked	100g	298	47.6	10.1	8.8
Oxtail, canned	100g	44	5.1	2.4	1.7
Oxtail, dried, cooked	100g	27	3.9	1.4	0.8
Tomato, dried, cooked	100g	31	6.3	0.6	0.5
Vegetable, canned, cooked	100g	37	6.7	1.5	0.7

Sweet and Savoury Snacks

Chocolate					
Aero	1 standard bar	252	26.7	4.0	14.4
Boost	1 bar [57g]	295	34.3	3.5	15.7
Bounty bar	1 mini bar [30g]	142	17.5	1.4	7.8
Caramac	1 standard bar [27g]	164	16.9	2.1	9.8
Chocolate cream	1 standard bar [50g]	215	36.3	1.4	6.9
Chocolate, milk	50g bar	265	29.7	4.2	15.2
Chocolate, plain	50g bar	263	32.4	2.4	14.6
Chocolate, white	50g bar	265	29.1	4.0	15.5
Creme egg	1 egg [39g]	150	22.6	1.6	6.6

Specific	Amount	Kcals	Carb	Prot	Fat
Crunchie	1 standard bar [42g]	195	30.5	1.9	8.0
Dairy Milk	1 medium bar [54g]	285	30.7	4.3	15.9
Flake	1 standard bar	170	19.9	2.8	9.7
Fudge	1 standard bar [30g]	130	21.6	1.0	5.2
Kit Kat	2 finger bar [20g]	100	12.1	1.6	5.3
Kit Kat	4 finger bar [50g]	250	30	0.8	2.7
Mars Bar	1 mini bar [20g]	88	13.3	1.1	3.8
Mars Bar	[68g]	300	9.0	0.7	2.6
Milky Bar	1 medium bar [20g]	110	11.1	1.7	6.4
Milky Way	1 standard size [55g]	218	34.8	2.4	8.7
Smarties	1 tube [36g]	164	26.6	1.9	6.3
Topic	1 bar [54g]	268	30.6	4.0	14.4
Turkish Delight	1 bar [51g]	190	37.8	0.8	3.9
Twirl	1 finger	115	12.3	1.8	6.6
Twix	50g bar	240	31.6	2.8	12.3
Non-chocolate confectionery					
Boiled sweets	100g	327	87.3	trace	trace
Fruit Gums	1 tube [33g]	57	14.8	0.3	0
Liquorice Allsorts	1 small bag [56g]	175	41.5	2.2	1.2
Starburst	1 pack [56g]	230	47.7	0.2	4.3
Pastilles, assorted	100g	253	61.9	5.2	0
Peppermints, assorted	100g	392	102.2	0.5	0.7
Popcorn, candied	100g	592	77.6	2.1	20.0
Popcorn, plain	100g	480	48.6	6.2	42.8
Skittles	1 pack [60g]	230	54.9	0.2	2.6
Toffees, mixed	100g	430	71.1	2.1	17.2
Turkish Delight	50g bar	198	38.9	0.3	0
Savoury Snacks					
Bombay mix	100g	503	35.1	18.8	32.9
Cheddars	100g	534	52.9	11.3	30.2
Corn snacks	100g	519	54.3	7.0	31.9
Peanuts and raisins	100g	435	37.5	15.3	26.0
Potato crisps, assorted	100g	546	49.3	5.6	37.6
Potato crisps, low-fat, assorted	100g	456	63.0	6.6	21.5
Potato Hoops	100g	523	58.5	3.9	32.0
Skips [KP]	100g	512	59.8	4.2	28.4
Skips [KP]	18g bag	92	10.8	0.8	5.1
Tortilla Chips	100g	459	60.1	7.6	22.6
Trail Mix	100g	432	37.2	9.1	28.5
Twiglets	100g	383	62.0	11.3	11.7
Wotsits	100g	545	52.4	9.4	33.1
Wotsits	21g bag	115	11.0	2.0	7.0

Alcoholic Drinks

Specific	Amount	Kcals	Carb	Prot	Fat
Ale					
bottled, brown	100ml	28	3	trace	nil
bottled, brown	1 pt	159	17	trace	nil
bottled, pale	100ml	32	2	trace	nil
bottled, pale	1 pt	182	11.4	trace	nil
strong	100ml	72	6.1	trace	nil
strong	1 pt	409	34.6	trace	nil
Beer					
bitter, canned	100ml	32	2.3	trace	nil
bitter, canned	1 pt	182	13.1	trace	nil
bitter, draught	100ml	32	2.3	trace	nil

Specific	Amount	Kcals	Carb	Prot	Fat
bitter, draught	1 pt	182	13.1	trace	nil
bitter, keg	100ml	31	2.3	trace	nil
bitter, keg	1 pt	177	13.1	trace	nil
mild, draught	100ml	25	1.6	trace	nil
mild, draught	1 pt	142	9.1	trace	nil
stout	100ml	37	4.2	trace	nil
stout	1 pt	210	23.5	trace	nil
stout, extra	100ml	39	2.1	trace	nil
stout, extra	1 pt	222	11.9	trace	nil
Cider					
dry	100ml	36	2.6	trace	nil
dry	1 pt	204	14.8	trace	nil
sweet	100ml	42	4.3	trace	nil
sweet	1 pt	238	24.4	trace	nil
vintage	100ml	101	7.3	trace	nil
vintage	1 pt	573	41.5	trace	nil
Fortified wine					
Port	30ml	47	3.6	trace	nil
Sherry, dry	30ml	35	0.5	trace	nil
Sherry, medium	30ml	35	1.0	trace	nil
Sherry, sweet	30ml	43	2	trace	nil
Lager					
bottled	100ml	29	1.5	trace	nil
bottled	1 pt	165	8.5	trace	nil
Spirits					
Brandy, 40% proof	30ml	65	trace	trace	nil
Gin, 40% proof	30ml	65	trace	trace	nil
Rum, 40% proof	30ml	65	trace	trace	nil
Vodka, 40% proof	30ml	65	trace	trace	nil
Whisky, 40% proof	30ml	65	trace	trace	nil
Wine					
red	100ml	68	0.3	trace	nil
red	1 glass [120ml]	82	0.4	trace	nil
rose, medium	100ml	71	2.5	trace	nil
rose, medium	1 glass [120ml]	853	3.0	trace	nil
white, dry	100ml	66	0.6	trace	nil
white, dry	1 glass [120ml]	79	0.7	trace	nil
white, medium	100ml	75	3.4	trace	nil
white, medium	1 glass [120ml]	90	4.1	trace	nil
white, sparkling	100ml	76	1.4	trace	nil
white, sparkling	1 glass [120ml]	91	1.7	trace	nil
white, sweet	100ml	94	5.9	trace	nil
white, sweet	1 glass [120ml]	113	53.2	trace	nil

Non-alcoholic Drinks

Specific	Amount	Kcals	Carb	Prot	Fat
Bournvita					
semi-skimmed milk	100g	58	7.8	3.5	1.6
whole milk	100g	76	7.6	3.4	3.8
powder	100g	341	79.0	7.7	1.5
Build-up					
semi-skimmed milk	100g	80	11.9	5.7	1.5
whole milk	100g	98	11.7	5.6	3.6
Carbonated drink					
Coca-cola	100g	36	10.5	trace	0
Coca-cola	can [330g]	119	5.0	trace	0

Specific	Amount	Kcals	Carb	Prot	Fat
Lemonade, bottled	100g	21	5.6	trace	0
Lucozade, bottled	100g	67	18.0	trace	0
Cocoa					
made with semi-skimmed milk	100g	57	7.0	3.5	1.9
made with whole milk	100g	76	6.8	3.4	4.2
powder	100g	312	11.5	18.5	21.7
Coffee					
instant, powder	100g	11.0	14.6	0	
instant, 30g of whole milk	1 mug	22	1.6	1.3	1.2
instant, without milk or sugar	1 mug [260g]	2	0.2	0.3	0
Coffeemate					
powder	100g	540	57.3	2.7	34.9
powder	portion [6g]	32	3.4	0.2	2.1
Complan					
sweet, water	100g	96	13.4	4.5	3.1
sweet, whole milk	100g	145	16.9	6.9	6.1
sweet, powder	100g	430	57.9	20.0	14.0
Cordial					
Lime juice cordial, undiluted	100g	112	29.8	0.1	0
Rosehip syrup, undiluted	100g	232	4.8	trace	0
Drinking chocolate					
made with semi-skimmed milk	100g	71	10.8	3.5	1.9
made with whole milk	100g	90	10.6	3.4	4.1
powder	100g	366	77.4	5.5	6.0
powder	1 mug [18g]	66	13.9	1.0	1.1
Horlicks					
instant, water	100g	51	10.1	2.4	0.5
made with semi-skimmed milk	100g	81	12.9	4.3	1.9
made with whole milk	100g	99	12.7	4.2	3.9
powder	100g	378	78.0	12.4	4.0
powder, low-fat, instant	100g	373	72.9	17.4	3.3
Juice					
Apple juice, unsweetened	100g	38	9.9	0.1	0.1
Grape juice, unsweetened	100g	46	11.7	0.3	0.1
Grapefruit juice, unsweetened	100g	33	8.3	0.4	0.1
Lemon juice, unsweetened	100g	7	1.6	0.3	trace
Orange juice, unsweetened	100g	36	8.8	0.5	0.1
Pineapple juice, unsweetened	100g	41	10.5	0.3	0.1
Tomato juice	100g	14	3.0	0.8	trace
Milk shake					
made with semi-skimmed milk	100g	69	11.3	3.2	1.6
made with whole milk	100g	87	11.1	3.1	3.7
powder	100g	388	98.3	1.3	1.6
thick, take-away	100g	90	13.2	2.9	3.2
Ovaltine					
made with semi-skimmed milk	100g	79	13.0	3.9	1.7
made with whole milk	100g	97	12.9	3.8	3.8
powder	100g	358	79.4	9.0	2.7
Squash					
Orange drink, undiluted	100g	107	28.5	trace	0
Ribena	100g	228	60.8	0.1	0
Tea					
no milk or sugar	100g	trace	trace	0.1	trace
no milk or sugar	1 cup [200g]	trace	trace	0.2	trace
with 30g of whole milk	1 cup [200g]	20	1.4	1.2	1.2

Fats and Oils

Animal fat

Compound cooking fat	100g	894	trace	trace	99.3
Dripping, beef	100g	891	trace	trace	99.0
Lard	100g	891	trace	trace	99.0
Suet, shredded	100g	826	12.1	trace	86.7

Ghee

Butter	100g	898	trace	trace	99.8
Palm	100g	897	trace	trace	99.7
Vegetable	100g	898	trace	trace	99.8

Oil

Coconut oil	100g	899	0	trace	99.9
Cod liver oil	100g	899	0	trace	99.9
Corn oil	100g	899	0	trace	99.9
Cottonseed oil	100g	899	0	trace	99.9
Olive oil	100g	899	0	trace	99.9
Palm oil	100g	899	0	trace	99.9
Peanut oil	100g	899	0	trace	99.9
Rapeseed oil	100g	899	0	trace	99.9
Safflower oil	100g	899	0	trace	99.9
Sesame oil	100g	881	0	0.2	99.7
Soya oil	100g	899	0	trace	99.9
Sunflower seed oil	100g	899	0	trace	99.9
Vegetable oil, blended, average	100g	899	0	trace	99.9
Wheatgerm oil	100g	899	0	trace	99.9

Spreading fat

Butter	100g	737	trace	0.5	81.7
Dairy/fat spread	100g	662	trace	0.4	73.4
Low-fat spread	100g	390	0.5	5.8	40.5
Margarine, hard, animal and vegetable fat	100g	739	1.0	0.2	81.6
Margarine, hard, vegetable fat only	100g	739	1.0	0.2	81.6
Margarine, soft, animal and vegetable fat	100g	739	1.0	0.2	81.6
Margarine, soft, vegetable fat only	100g	739	1.0	0.2	81.6
Margarine, polyunsaturated	100g	739	1.0	0.2	81.6
Very low-fat spread	100g	273	3.6	8.3	25.0

Preserves

Jam, fruit	100g	261	69.0	0.6	0
Jam, stone fruit	100g	261	69.3	0.4	0
Jam, reduced sugar	100g	123	31.9	0.5	0
Lemon curd	100g	283	62.7	0.6	5.1
Marmalade	100g	261	69.5	0.1	0
Mincemeat	100g	274	62.1	0.6	4.3

Spread

Chocolate and nut	100g	549	60.5	6.2	33.0
Honey	100g	288	76.4	0.4	0
Honey and comb	100g	281	74.4	0.6	4.6

Sugar

Demerara	100g	394	104.5	0.5	0
Glucose liquid	100g	318	84.7	trace	0
White sugar	100g	394	105.0	trace	0
Syrup, golden	100g	298	79.0	0.3	0
Treacle, black	100g	257	67.2	1.2	0